Controlling Gestational Diabetes

The Sugar Diet Control

By

Angel Burns

License Notices

This book or parts thereof might not be reproduced in any format for personal or commercial use without the written permission of the author. Possession and distribution of this book by any means without said permission is prohibited by law.

All content is for entertainment purposes and the author accepts no responsibility for any damages, commercially or personally, caused by following the content.

Get Your Daily Deals Here!

Free books on me! Subscribe now to receive free and discounted books directly to your email. This means you will always have choices of your next book from the comfort of your own home and a reminder email will pop up a few days beforehand, so you never miss out! Every day, free books will make their way into your inbox and all you need to do is choose what you want.

What could be better than that?

Fill out the box below to get started on this amazing offer and start receiving your daily deals right away!

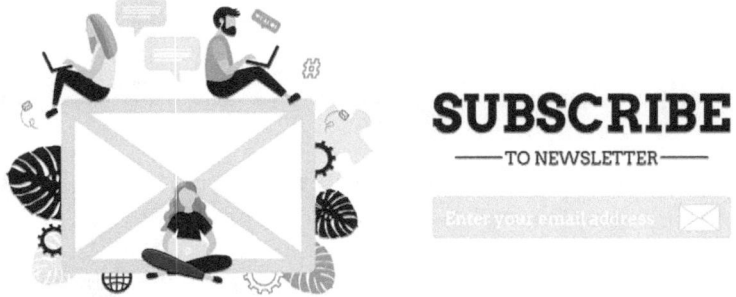

https://angel-burns.gr8.com

Table of Contents

Gestational Diabetes Recipes

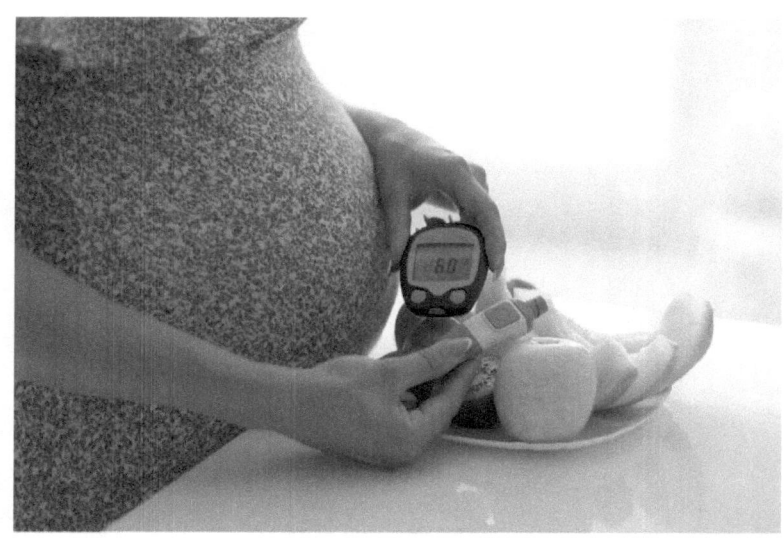

Chapter I – Snack Ideas

HHHHHHHHHHHHHHHHHHHHHHHHHHHHHHHHHHHH

Recipe 1: Coconut Almond Cookies

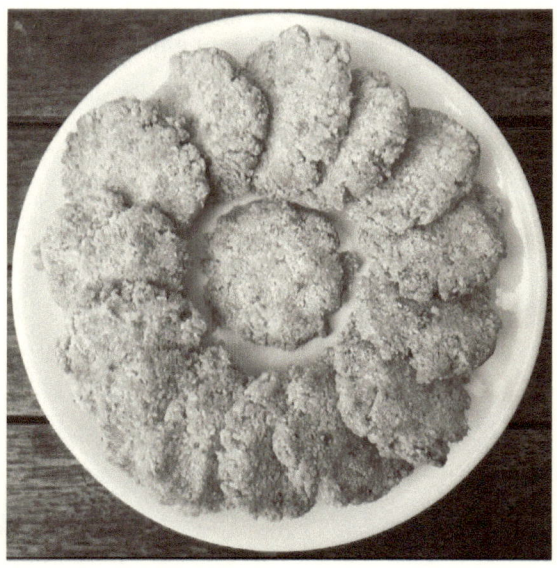

There is no one who can refuse the delicacy of this cookie. The collaboration of almond and cheese, serve tasty cookies that can make your tongue dance. Once you have spare time, make this cookie in double or more portions then store in a jar with lid. Enjoy a serving of this special cookie in your snack time.

Yield: 2

Preparation Time: 25 minutes

Ingredient List:

- ½ cup almond butter
- ¼ cup grated cheese
- 2 egg yolks
- 1 cup almond flour
- ½ cup coconut flakes

HHHHHHHHHHHHHHHHHHHHHHHHHHHHHHHHHHHH

Procedure:

1. Preheat an oven to 250°F then line a baking sheet with a parchment paper.

2. Place almond butter in a mixing bowl then add egg yolks to it. Using an electric mixer whisk until combined and smooth.

3. Add grated cheese to the butter mixture then whisk again until incorporated.

4. Next, stir in almond flour then using a wooden spatula mix until becoming dough.

5. After that, add coconut flakes to your dough and then mix until just combined.

6. Shape the dough into small balls then press each ball until becoming coin.

7. Arrange the coins on the prepared baking sheet and then bake for about 20 minutes or until the top of the cookies are lightly golden.

8. Once it is done, move from the oven to a cooling rack.

9. When the cookies are cool, store in a jar with a lid then enjoy anytime you want.

Each serving contains 143 Calories, 1.1 g Sugar, 3.8 g Net Carbs, 12.6 g Fats, 5.4 g Protein

Recipe 2: Simple Roasted Squash

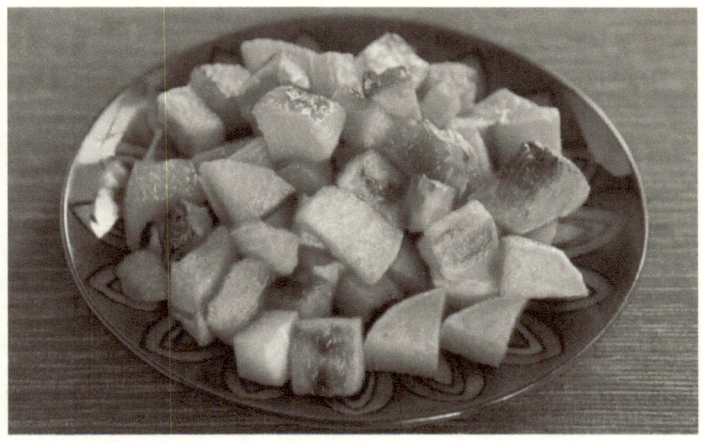

Almost all women do lots of efforts to beautify their skin and hair including a pregnant woman. Butternut squash is a kind of vegetables that promises to nourish your skin and hair. The high content of vitamin C in butternut squash helps you to moisturize your skin, delay wrinkles, and stimulate hair growth. Especially for a pregnant woman, butternut squash helps to develop the baby's brain and spinal cord. The butternut squash gives more opportunity for a pregnant woman to deliver a healthy baby.

Yield: 2

Preparation Time: 45 minutes

Ingredient List:

- ½ lb. butternut squash cubes
- ¾ tbsp. olive oil
- ¼ tsp. cumin
- 2 tbsp. almond butter

HHHHHHHHHHHHHHHHHHHHHHHHHHHHHHHHHHH

Procedure:

1. Preheat an oven to 400°F then line a baking sheet with a parchment paper.

2. Microwave the almond butter until melted then combine with olive oil and cumin.

3. Peel the butternut squash then cut into wedges.

4. Toss the butternut squash with the butter mixture then spread on the prepared baking sheet.

5. Roast your butternut squash for approximately 30 minutes or until the squash is tender.

6. Once it is done, remove from the oven then transfer to a serving dish.

7. Serve and enjoy.

Each serving contains 197 Calories, 3.4 g Sugar, 16.5 g Net Carbs, 14.3 g Fats, 4.8 g Protein

Recipe 3: Unsweetened Roasted Cashew

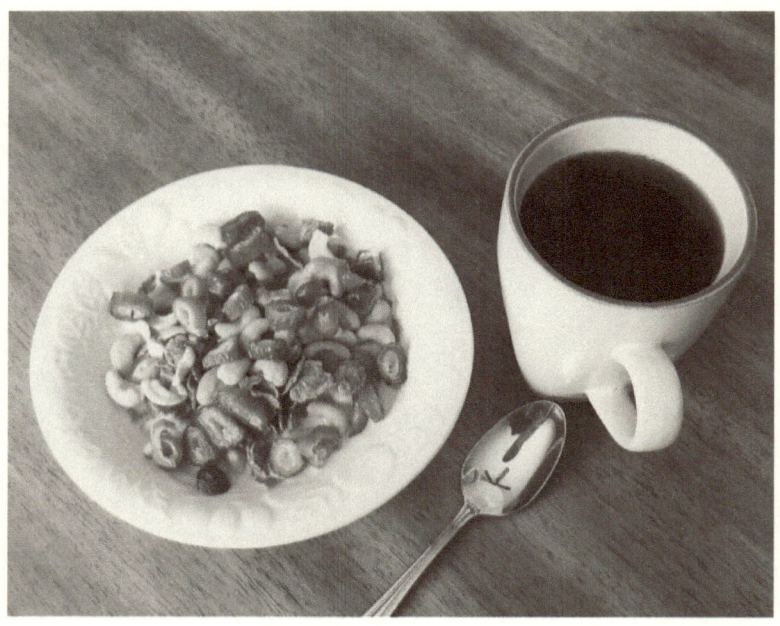

Unless you have an allergy to this nut, cashew is okay to be consumed during your pregnancy. There is no doubt that cashew is the best source of protein and fats among other nuts. Besides that, it is also high in fiber, iron, vitamin K, and magnesium that are great for an expectant mother. However, eating too much cashew may cause weight gain. So, have this snack in moderation is best.

Yield: 4

Preparation Time: 15 minutes

Ingredient List:

- ¾ cup raw cashew
- ½ tsp. olive oil

HHHHHHHHHHHHHHHHHHHHHHHHHHHHHHHHHHHHH

Procedure:

1. Preheat an oven to 375°F then line a baking sheet with parchment paper.

2. Spread the cashew on the prepared baking sheet and then bake for 15 minutes.

3. Stirring the cashew every 5 minutes. Pay attention to the doneness of the cashew because it can be quickly burnt.

4. Once the cashew is done, remove from the oven then drizzle olive oil over the cashew. Toss to combine.

5. Transfer to a serving dish or jar then enjoy in your movie time.

Each serving contains 153 Calories, 1.3 g Sugar, 8.4 g Net Carbs, 12.5 g Fats, 3.9 g Protein

Recipe 4: The Berries Muffin

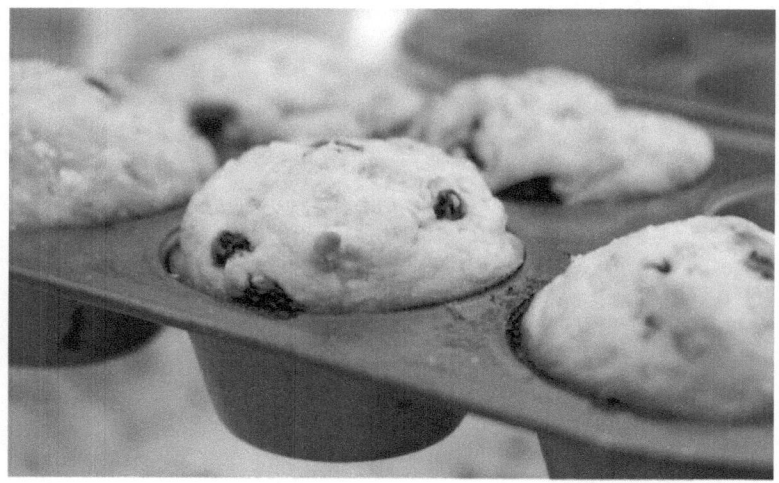

A pregnant woman can eat this low-sugar berry muffin without feeling guilty. Berry, for sure, is not only safe but also good for a pregnant woman. It contains potassium that is essential to control the blood pressure. So, it can be said that berry helps the pregnant woman to reduce the risk of having preeclampsia.

Yield: 4

Preparation Time: 30 minutes

Ingredient List:

- ¼ cup coconut oil
- 2 organic eggs
- 1 cup almond yogurt
- 1 tsp. orange zest
- 1-½ cups almond flour
- ¾ tsp. cinnamon
- ¼ cup chopped blueberries
- ¼ cup chopped cranberries

HHHHHHHHHHHHHHHHHHHHHHHHHHHHHHHHHH

Procedure:

1. Preheat an oven to 375°F then prepare 8 paper muffin cups. Set aside.

2. Place almond flour in a bowl then add orange zest and cinnamon. Mix well.

3. Crack the organic eggs then place in another bowl. Stir until just beaten.

4. Pour coconut oil and almond yogurt into the beaten eggs then mix until incorporated.

5. Pour the liquid mixture over the dry mixture then stir until combined.

6. Add chopped blueberries and cranberries into the mixture then divide into the prepared muffin cups.

7. Bake the muffins for approximately 20 minutes or until a stick inserted comes out clean.

8. Once it is done, remove from the oven then place on a cooling rack.

9. Transfer the muffins to a serving platter then serve.

10. Enjoy!

Each serving contains 252 Calories, 4.7 g Sugar, 11.6 g Net Carbs, 21.8 g Fats, 5.4 g Protein

Recipe 5: Almond Egg Tart

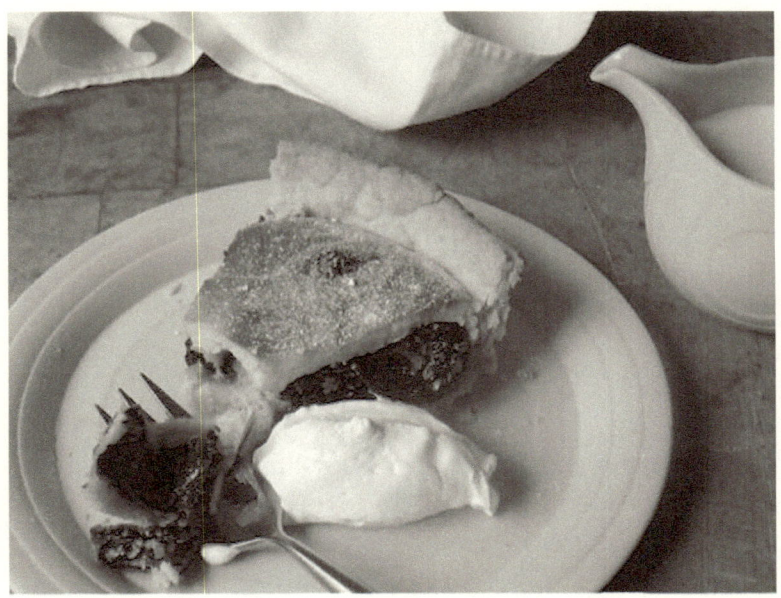

This almond tart is very easy to make. Being very low in sugar, this snack can be a right option for you during your pregnancy. The filling, which is so soft and smooth, gives additional sensation for this snack. As a variant, you can add any ingredients that are available in your refrigerator. Meat, mushroom, or vegetable can be added to enhance the taste and the healthy content of this dish. Enjoy!

Yield: 4

Preparation Time: 45 minutes

Ingredient List:

- ½ cup almond flour
- ¼ cup almond butter
- 1 organic egg yolk
- 3 organic eggs
- ¼ cup almond milk

HHHHHHHHHHHHHHHHHHHHHHHHHHHHHHHHHHHHH

Procedure:

1. Place butter and egg yolk in a bowl then beat to combine.

2. When the butter is smooth, add almond flour to the bowl. Using a wooden spatula, mix well.

3. Preheat an oven to 350°F then coat 10 small pie pans with butter or oil.

4. Divide the dough into ten then fill each pan with a part of dough. Press the dough into the pan.

5. Bake the pies for 10 minutes until the top of the pies are lightly golden.

6. Take the pies out from the oven then let them cool for a few minutes.

7. Reduce the heat of the oven.

8. Meanwhile, crack the eggs then place in a bowl.

9. Pour milk into the eggs then whisk until incorporated.

10. Fill each pie with the egg mixture then bake again for about 10-15 minutes or until the egg mixture is set.

11. Once it is done, remove from the oven and let the pies cool.

12. Take the pies out from the pan then arrange on a serving dish.

13. Serve and enjoy.

Each serving contains 243 Calories, 1.9 g Sugar, 4.4 g Net Carbs, 20.6 g Fats, 12.3 g Protein

Recipe 6: Coconut Squares

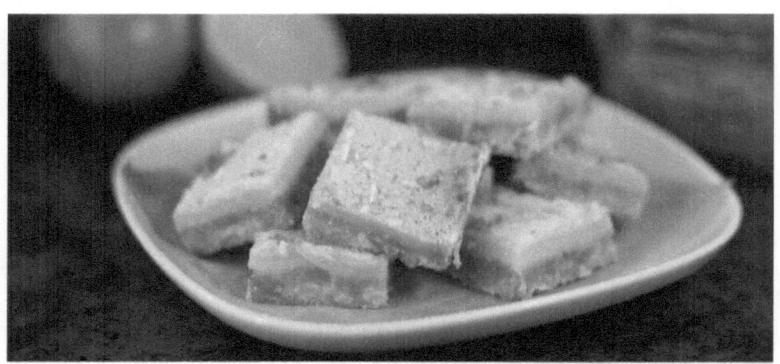

Coconut provides fatty acids that are necessary for the baby's brain development. It is also a source of energy without increasing the blood sugar level like carbohydrates do. Because coconut is also low in sugar, it prevents a pregnant woman from a morning sickness that is always annoying. Involving coconut in your snack time is really a right option.

Yield: 2

Preparation Time: 20 minutes

Ingredient List:

- 1 cup shredded coconut
- 2 tbsp. coconut butter
- 2 organic eggs

Procedure:

1. Preheat an oven to 350°F then line a baking sheet with aluminum foil.

2. Melt the coconut oil then combine with eggs. Stir until incorporated.

3. Add shredded coconut to the mixture then mix well.

4. Transfer the mixture to the prepared baked sheet then spread evenly.

5. Bake for approximately 10 minutes then remove from heat. Place on the cooling rack.

6. Once it warm, cut into squares then transfer to a serving dish.

7. Serve and enjoy.

Each serving contains 260 Calories, 3.3 g Sugar, 8.4 g Net Carbs, 23 g Fats, 7.4 g Protein

Recipe 7: Coconut Chicken Crispy

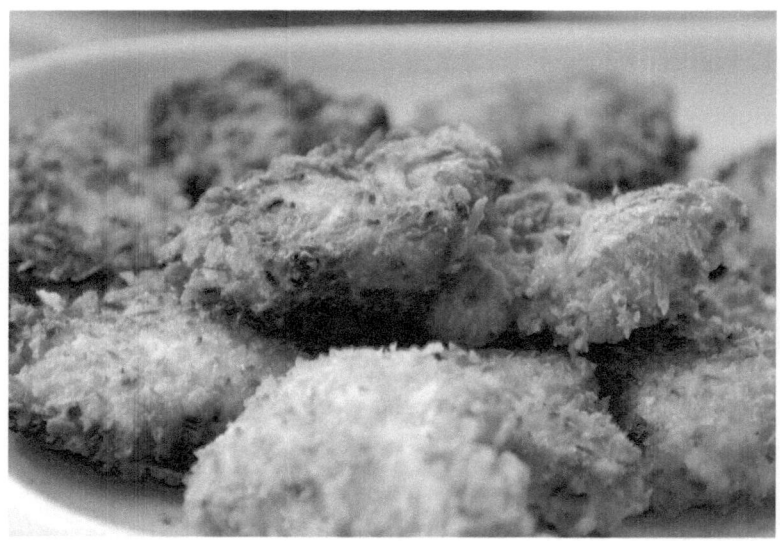

Who can say no to crispy chicken? It has become almost all people favorite's choice of go-to food. Unlike other crispy chicken that is high in carbs, this dish is low in carbs. If you don't have chicken is not available, you can change it with fish. It will also taste great.

Yield: 4

Preparation Time: 45 minutes

Ingredient List:

- ½ lb. chicken fillet
- 2 organic eggs
- 3 tbsp. coconut flour
- ¼ cup coconut flakes
- ½ tsp. pepper

HHHHHHHHHHHHHHHHHHHHHHHHHHHHHHHHHHH

Procedure:

1. Preheat an oven to 350°F then line a baking pan with parchment paper.

2. Crack the eggs then place in a bowl.

3. Season with pepper then beat until incorporated.

4. Place coconut flakes and coconut flour in two different bowls.

5. Cut the chicken into slices then place in a plate.

6. Take a slice of chicken then dip in the egg mixture.

7. Roll the chicken in the coconut flour, dip again in the egg mixture then roll in the coconut flakes.

8. Place the coated chicken in the prepared baking pan then repeat with the remaining chicken.

9. Bake the chicken for about 20 minutes or until your chicken crispy is brown.

10. Once it is done, remove from the oven then transfer to a serving dish.

11. Serve and enjoy immediately.

Each serving contains 250 Calories, 3.1 g Sugar, 10.2 g Net Carbs, 15.3 g Fats, 18.2 g Protein

Recipe 8: Avocado and Strawberry Salads

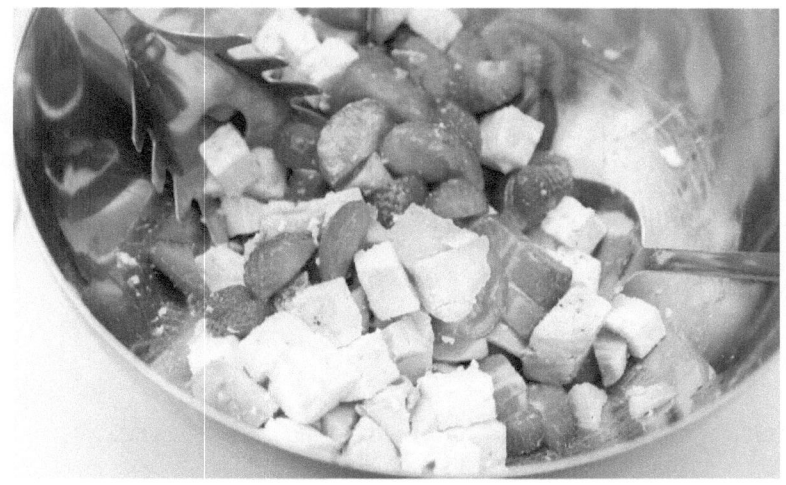

Both avocado and strawberry are good to be consumed by a pregnant woman. With a high amount of folic acid, avocado and strawberry strengthen the baby's nerves and decrease the risk of having baby with disabilities. For the best result, always choose ripe avocado and strawberry.

Yield: 2

Preparation Time: 15 minutes

Ingredient List:

- 1 ripe avocado
- ½ cup fresh strawberries
- 1 cup chopped fresh lettuce
- 3 tsp. lemon juice
- 2 tsp. cider vinegar
- 3 tsp. olive oil

HHHHHHHHHHHHHHHHHHHHHHHHHHHHHHHHHHHHH

Procedure:

1. Cut the avocado into halves then discard the seed.

2. Scoop out the avocado flesh then place in a salad bowl.

3. Cut the strawberries into halves or quarters then add to the same bowl with avocado.

4. Add chopped fresh lettuce into the bowl then drizzle lemon juice, cider vinegar, and olive oil over the salad ingredients. Toss to combine.

5. Serve and enjoy.

Each serving contains 283 Calories, 2.7 g Sugar, 12.5 g Net Carbs, 26.8 g Fats, 2.3 g Protein

Recipe 9: Meaty Tofu Bars

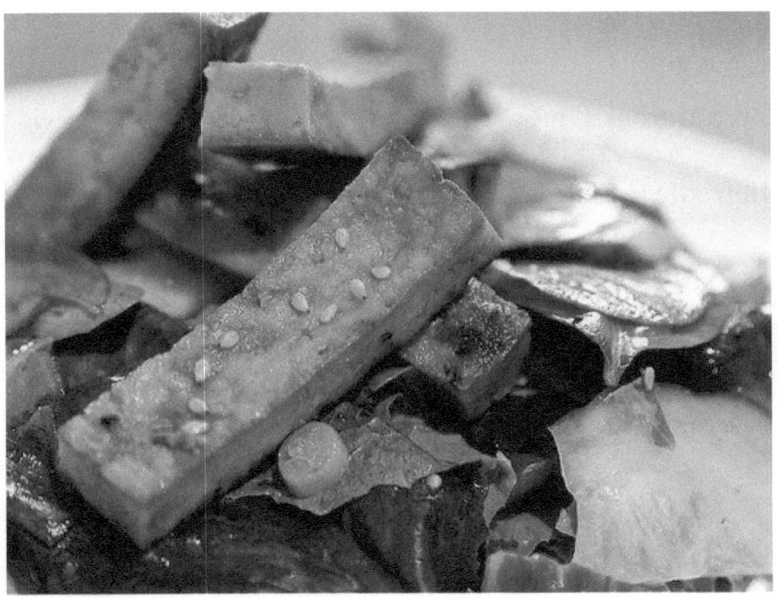

It can be denied that tofu is rich in essential nutrients that are needed in pregnancy. Being low in calorie, tofu is a great choice of food for a pregnant woman because it is also rich in amino acid. Consuming amino acid in moderation is recommended to a pregnant woman for it will reduce the risk of having preeclampsia. This dish is a delicious and easy to make food that you can eat in your snacking time. With additional ingredients such as eggs and meat, this dish surely becomes a great source of protein. For a healthier variation, you can include vegetable to this dish like carrot, leek, or spinach.

Yield: 4

Preparation Time: 45 minutes

Ingredient List:

- 1 lb. firm tofu
- 4 organic eggs
- ½ cup ground beef
- 2 tsp. minced garlic
- ½ tsp. pepper

HHHHHHHHHHHHHHHHHHHHHHHHHHHHHHHHHHHHH

Procedure:

1. Preheat a steamer over medium heat then coat a heatproof pan with cooking spray. The pan must fit to the steamer.

2. Place the entire ingredients in a food processor then process until smooth.

3. Transfer the mixture to the prepared pan then spread evenly.

4. Place the pan in the steamer then steam for about 20 minutes until the tofu mixture is firm.

5. When the tofu is done, remove from the steamer and let it cool.

6. Cut the cooked tofu into bars form then set aside.

7. Preheat an oven to 350°F then lines a baking sheet with aluminum foil.

8. Arrange then tofu bars on the prepared baking sheet then bake for about 5 minutes or until the tofu bars are lightly golden.

9. When the tofu is done, transfer to a serving dish.

10. Serve and enjoy.

Each serving contains 291 Calories, 2.1 g Sugar, 5.8 g Net Carbs, 18.3 g Fats, 30 g Protein

Recipe 10: Cheesy Spinach Balls

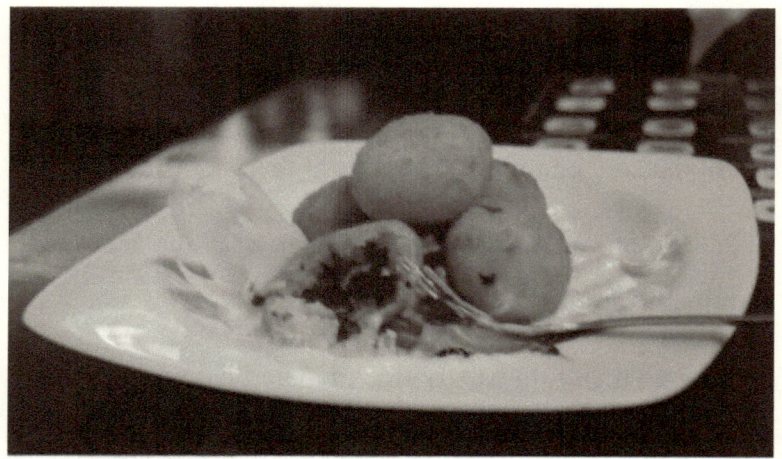

If you are looking for a kind of vegetable that is not only healthy but also tasty, why don't you choose spinach? Spinach, which is known as a great source of folic acid, is good for a pregnant woman for it decreases the risk of having anemia and premature birth. This vegetable is not only perfect for lunch or dinner but also for snack. These balls, which use spinach as the main ingredients is the right choice to accompany your snack time. Some people love to enjoy these spinach balls with savory coconut milk.

Yield: 2

Preparation Time: 15 minutes

Ingredient List:

- 3 cups chopped spinach
- ½ cup almond flour
- ¼ cup grated cheese
- 2 tbsp. chopped leek
- 3 organic eggs
- 1 ½ tbsp. almond butter, melted
- ½ tsp. pepper

HHHHHHHHHHHHHHHHHHHHHHHHHHHHHHHHHHHH

Procedure:

1. Preheat an oven to 350°F then line a baking sheet with parchment paper.

2. Combine all ingredients in a bowl then mix well.

3. Shape the mixture into balls form then arrange on the prepared baking sheet.

4. Bake the spinach balls for about 15 minutes until the spinach balls are done.

5. Remove from the oven then transfer to a serving dish.

6. Serve and enjoy.

Each serving contains 280 Calories, 1.8 g Sugar, 17.2 g Net Carbs, 21.7 g Fats, 17.3 g Protein

Chapter II – Breakfast Ideas

HHHHHHHHHHHHHHHHHHHHHHHHHHHHHHHHHHHHH

Recipe 11: Spinach Mushroom Quiche

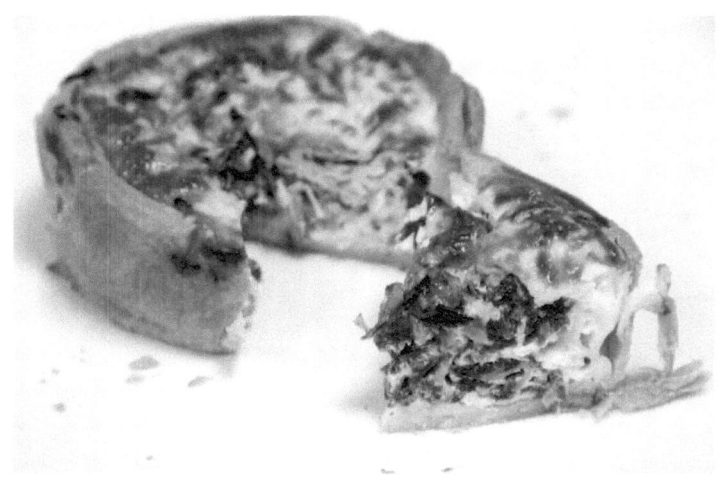

Who doesn't like quiche? With some spinach and mushroom as the source of zinc, potassium, irons, folate, magnesium, and antioxidant, this dish is perfect nutrition for both the mom and the baby. Please make sure that you choose particular kind of cheese that is pasteurized, which is mainly found in the hard cheese section at your local store.

Yield: 2

Preparation Time: 50 minutes

Ingredient List:

- 1 cup chopped spinach
- ½ cup chopped mushroom
- 4 organic eggs
- ¾ tbsp. olive oil
- ¼ cup chopped onion
- ¼ cup grated cheese
- ¼ tsp. black pepper

HHHHHHHHHHHHHHHHHHHHHHHHHHHHHHHHHHH

Procedure:

1. Preheat an oven to 350°F then grease a medium pie pan with cooking spray. Set aside.

2. Preheat a skillet over medium heat then pour olive oil into it.

3. When the oil is hot, stir in chopped onion and sauté until wilted and aromatic.

4. Next, add spinach and mushroom to the skillet then stir until just wilted. Remove from heat.

5. Crack the eggs then place in a bowl.

6. Add cheese and pepper to the eggs then whisk until beaten.

7. Stir in the spinach and mushroom into the eggs then mix well.

8. Transfer the mixture to the prepared pie pan then spread evenly.

9. Bake for about 30 minutes or until the quiche is set.

10. When the quiche is done, remove from the oven then let it cool for 3-4 minutes.

11. Serve and enjoy.

Each serving contains 179 Calories, 3.5 g Sugar, 11.9 g Net Carbs, 14.4 g Fats, 1.2 g Protein

Recipe 12: Almond Berry Porridge

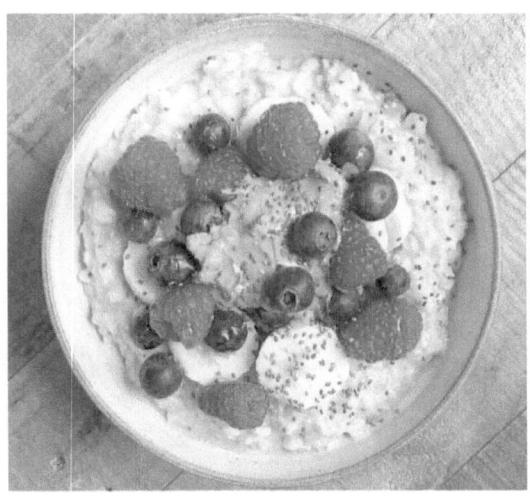

As breakfast is the most important meal of the day, you have to be careful in choosing the right amount of food you eat at this particular time. You need a few carbs to fuel your body with overflowing energy to go through the day, as well as vitamins, protein, and minerals. The combination of the overall ingredients in this porridge is a great way to start your day. You can choose other fruits of your favorite. You can also add some other source of plant-based protein in some nuts other than almond.

Yield: 1

Preparation Time: 5 Minutes

Ingredient List:

- ¼ cup almond flour
- 1 tbsp. flax seeds
- ¾ cup water
- 1 organic egg
- 1 tbsp. almond butter
- ¼ cup mixed fresh strawberries and blueberries

HHHHHHHHHHHHHHHHHHHHHHHHHHHHHHHHHHHHH

Procedure:

1. Combine almond flour and flax seeds in a saucepan then pour water over the mixture. Stir well then bring to a simmer.

2. Once the mixture starts to simmer, reduce the heat then whisk until the mixture is thickened. Remove from heat then set aside.

3. Crack the organic eggs then place in a bowl. Using a fork stir the eggs until beaten then pour it over the almond flour mixture. Mix well.

4. Return the porridge to heat then stir for about a half an hour or until incorporated.

5. Stir in almond butter and coconut milk then mix well. Remove from heat.

6. Transfer the almond porridge to four serving bowls then garnish with fresh strawberries and blueberries on top.

7. Serve and enjoy immediately.

Each serving contains 250 Calories, 3.3 g Sugar, 9.8 g Net Carbs, 19.2 g Fats, 12 g Protein

Recipe 13: Baked Sweet Potato

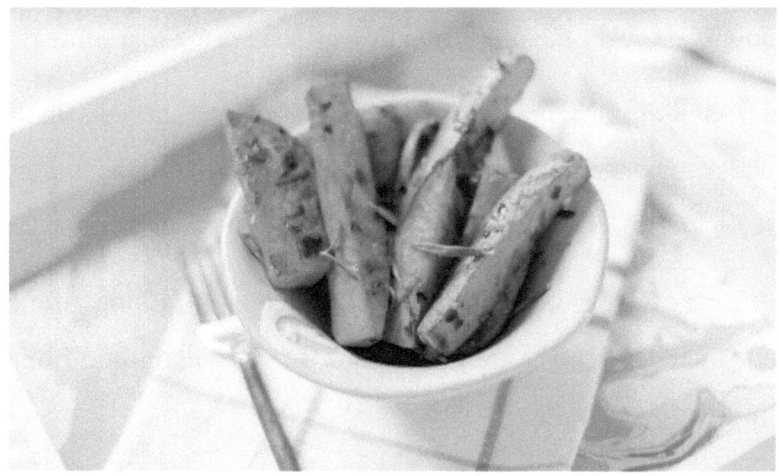

Nutrition has become a priority for a pregnant woman. Sweet potato is a great choice to support the pregnancy for it contains high nutrients. As an excellent source of beta-carotene, sweet potato is an excellent food to be consumed by a pregnant woman. Furthermore, the fiber content in this food improves the digestive system and encourages it to run better.

Yield: 2

Preparation Time: 55 minutes

Ingredient List:

- 2 medium sweet potatoes
- 2 ½ tbsp. butter
- ½ tsp. pepper

HHHHHHHHHHHHHHHHHHHHHHHHHHHHHHHHHHHHH

Procedure:

1. Preheat an oven to 425°F then prepare a baking sheet.

2. Using a fork prick the sweet potatoes on all sides.

3. Place the sweet potatoes on the prepared baking dish then bake for approximately 50 minutes.

4. Once it is done, remove the sweet potatoes from the oven then using a knife split the sweet potatoes.

5. Top with butter and wait until it is melted.

6. Serve and enjoy immediately.

Each serving contains 179 Calories, 3.5 g Sugar, 11.9 g Net Carbs, 14.4 g Fats, 1.2 g Protein

Recipe 14: Cheesy Omelet with Tomato

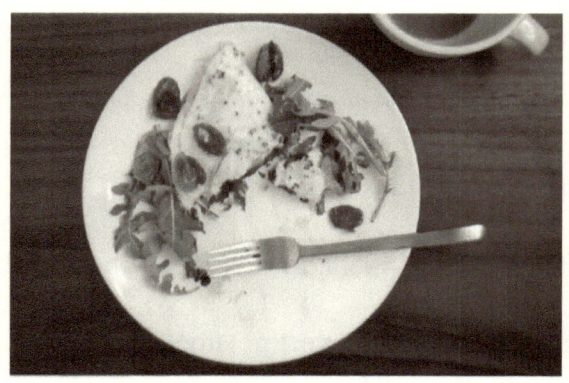

Pregnant women will feel extremely hungry in the morning because they don't eat for more than 8 hours when they sleep. If you don't have lots of time in the morning, this omelet can be an alternative to breakfast. With the presence of cheese and tomato, this more than just a regular omelet. It will be a healthy and nutritious breakfast of the day. For higher nutrient content, you can add other nutritious ingredients such as mushroom, meat, or vegetables if you wish.

Yield: 1

Preparation Time: 5 Minutes

Ingredient List:

- 2 organic eggs
- ¼ tsp. pepper
- 1-tsp. olive oil
- 2 tbsp. grated Mozzarella cheese
- 2 tbsp. diced tomato

HHHHHHHHHHHHHHHHHHHHHHHHHHHHHHHHHHH

Procedure:

1. Crack the eggs then place in a bowl.

2. Season the eggs with pepper then whisk until fully incorporated.

3. Preheat a pan over medium heat then pour olive oil into the pan.

4. Once the oil is hot, pour the egg mixture over the pan then make an omelet.

5. When the omelet is done, transfer to baking pan.

6. Sprinkle the grated mozzarella cheese over the omelet then bake the omelet for a few seconds in a preheated oven.

7. Remove from the oven then sprinkle diced tomato on top.

8. Serve and enjoy immediately.

Each serving contains 331 Calories, 1.3 g Sugar, 3.9 g Net Carbs, 23.5 g Fats, 27.3 g Protein

Recipe 15: Cheesy Vegetable Frittata

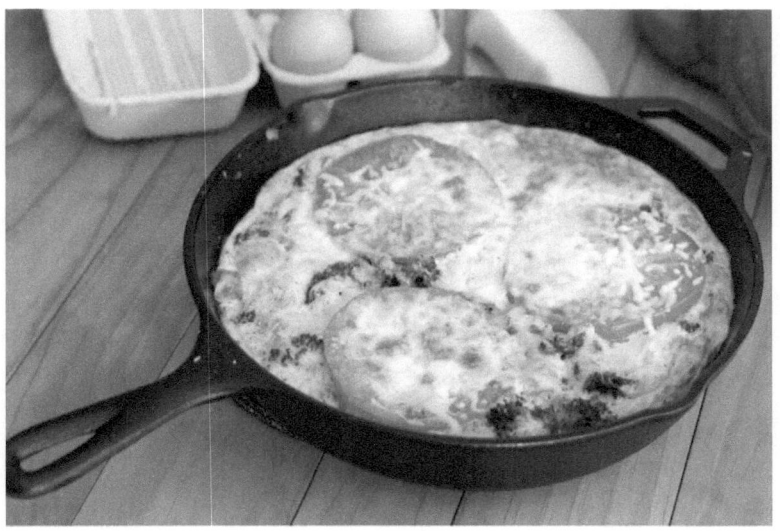

This frittata is a great way to combine protein in eggs with vitamins and minerals in vegetables. Not only broccoli and spinach, you can also add cauliflower, carrot, and kale if you wish. Those kinds of vegetables provide good nutrients for your pregnancy. Another benefit of cooking this frittata is that it is not only good for a pregnant woman but also for the whole family. Besides, serving delicious breakfast with high nutrients for your family, you also save your time.

Yield: 2

Preparation Time: 15 minutes

Ingredient List:

- 4 organic eggs
- 3 organic egg whites
- 1 cup chopped broccoli
- 1-½ tsp. water
- 1 cup chopped spinach
- 1 ½ tsp. olive oil
- ¼ cup chopped onion
- 1 tsp. minced garlic
- ¼ tsp. black pepper
- ¼ cup grated cheese

HHHHHHHHHHHHHHHHHHHHHHHHHHHHHHHHHHH

Procedure:

1. Preheat an oven to 400°F.

2. Preheat an oven-safe non-stick pan over medium heat then pour olive oil into it.

3. Once the oil is hot, stir in minced garlic and chopped onion then sauté until aromatic.

4. Add spinach and broccoli to the pan then cook until just wilted. Remove from heat.

5. Crack the eggs then place in a bowl.

6. Add egg whites and water then season with pepper. Mix well.

7. Pour the egg mixture over the pan then sprinkle grated cheese on top.

8. Bake the frittata for approximately 10 minutes or until the eggs are set.

9. Once it is done, remove from the oven then let it cool for about 5 minutes.

10. Cut into wedges then serve.

11. Enjoy.

Each serving contains 266 Calories, 2.6 g Sugar, 6.8 g Net Carbs, 17.3 g Fats, 22 g Protein

Recipe 16: Easy Coconut Granola

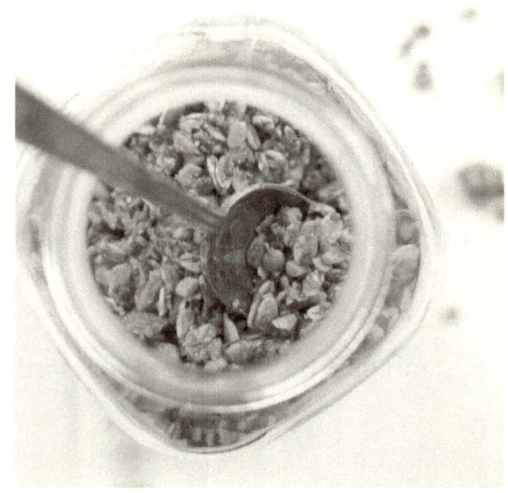

Why should you buy prepackaged granola if you can create it yourself? Not only it is healthier, preservative free, and other artificial ingredients-free, it also has less sugar. Prepare the ingredients as instructed and serve with some plant-based milk.

Yield: 2

Preparation Time: 45 Minutes

Ingredient List:

- 1-½ cups rolled oats
- ½ cup shredded coconut
- 3 tbsp. chopped peanut
- 3 tbsp. chopped walnut
- 1 tbsp. flax seeds
- ½ tbsp. canola oil
- ¾ tsp. cinnamon

HHHHHHHHHHHHHHHHHHHHHHHHHHHHHHHHHHHH

Procedure:

1. Preheat an oven to 300°F then lines a baking sheet with parchment paper.

2. Combine oats with shredded coconut, walnut, cashew, and flax seeds in a bowl. Mix well.

3. Drizzle canola oil and cinnamon over the mixture then toss to combine.

4. Spread the mixture on the prepared baking sheet then bake for approximately 45 minutes or until the nuts and seeds are crunchy.

5. Once it is done, store the granola in a jar with a lid.

6. Enjoy with almond milk or coconut milk.

Each serving contains 214 Calories, 1.2 g Sugar, 17.9 g Net Carbs, 13.8 g Fats, 6.5 g Protein

Recipe 17: Quinoa and Peach Porridge

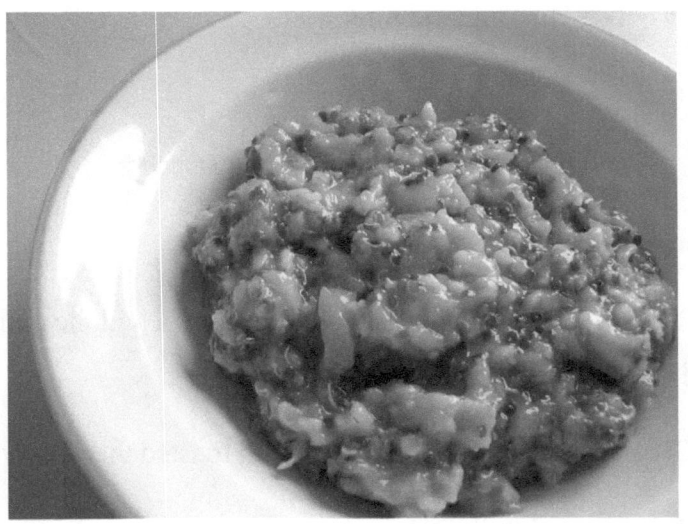

If you are looking for a delicious but simple breakfast, this quinoa porridge may be the right answer. Quinoa is known as a superfood with unprocessed whole grain. Besides that, quinoa is rich in magnesium that is needed by a pregnant woman to prevent premature contraction. Enjoy this quinoa porridge just the way it is or top with fresh fruits or roasted nuts.

Yield: 2

Preparation Time: 35 minutes

Ingredient List:

- ¾ cup quinoa
- ½ tsp. cinnamon
- 1-¾ cups almond milk
- ¾ cup water

HHHHHHHHHHHHHHHHHHHHHHHHHHHHHHHHHHHH

Procedure:

1. Preheat a saucepan over medium heat then add the quinoa and cinnamon into it.

2. Cook the quinoa and cinnamon until toasted then stir well.

3. Pour almond milk and water into the saucepan then bring to boil.

4. Once it is boiled, reduce the heat then cook until thick.

5. When the quinoa porridge is done, transfer to a serving bowl.

6. Serve and enjoy.

Each serving contains 195 Calories, 3.8 g Sugar, 32.7 g Net Carbs, 4.2 g Fats, 6.7 g Protein

Recipe 18: Soft Almond Pancakes

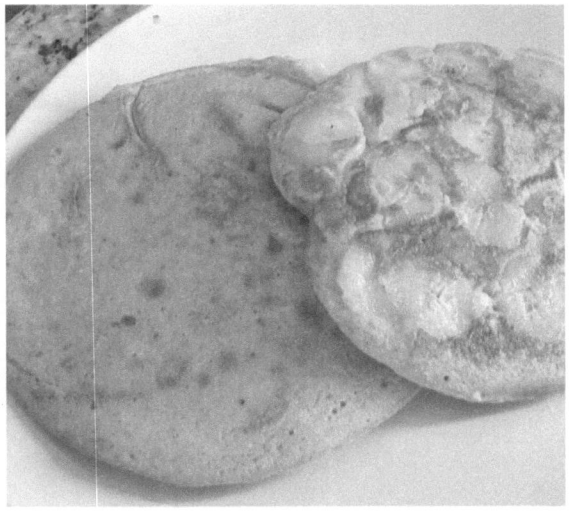

Pancake that is made from almond flour is gluten-free. This is why; this pancake recipe is a great choice for you who are watching your carbs intake. Since this pancake is low carbs, surely, it becomes a perfect choice for a pregnant woman with gestational diabetes. In addition, this pancake helps you to enjoy delicious pancake without worrying the increase of blood sugar level.

Yield: 1

Preparation Time: 5 minutes

Ingredient List:

- 1 organic egg
- 1 tsp. almond oil
- ½ cup unsweetened almond yogurt
- 1-tbsp. almond flour

HHHHHHHHHHHHHHHHHHHHHHHHHHHHHHHHHHH

Procedure:

1. Place almond flour in a blender then pour almond yogurt into it.

2. Crack the egg then place in the blender. Blend until smooth and incorporated.

3. Preheat a pan over medium heat then brush the pan with almond oil.

4. Pour about two tbsp. of batter into the pan then cook for about a minute.

5. Flip the pancake then cook until both sides of the pancakes are lightly golden.

6. Transfer pancake to a serving dish then repeat with the remaining ingredients.

7. Serve and enjoy.

Each serving contains 208 Calories, 5.5 g Sugar, 10.6 g Net Carbs, 15.1 g Fats, 8.3 g Protein

Recipe 19: Healthy and Meaty Sweet Potato Casserole

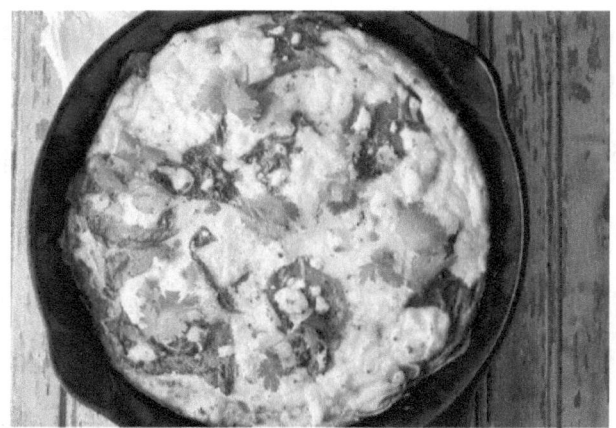

Casserole is a friendly comfort food for busy people. It can be prepared ahead with flexible ingredients. However, for a pregnant woman, the ingredients for the casserole should meet all the nutritional needs she and her baby needs. This casserole provides carbs from sweet potato, protein from cheese and eggs, and vitamins from the vegetables. For an extra delicacy, you can also add meat and other herbs. Prepare this casserole the night before and microwave it in the morning.

Yield: 4

Preparation Time: 1 hour

Ingredient List:

- 1-½ cups sliced sweet potato
- ¾ cup ground beef
- 1 cup chopped broccoli
- ½ cup chopped onion
- 2 tsp. minced garlic
- ½ cup grated Mozzarella cheese
- 1-½ tbsp. Dijon mustard
- ½ cup coconut milk
- 3 organic eggs

HHHHHHHHHHHHHHHHHHHHHHHHHHHHHHHHH

Procedure:

1. Preheat an oven to 350°F then coat a baking dish with cooking spray.

2. Arrange sliced sweet potato in the bottom of a baking dish then sprinkle chopped broccoli, chopped onion, and ground beef over the sweet potato. Set aside.

3. Crack the eggs then place in a bowl.

4. Season with minced garlic and Dijon mustard then pour coconut milk into the eggs. Whisk until incorporated.

5. Pour the egg mixture over the sliced potato then sprinkle grated Mozzarella cheese on top.

6. Cover the sweet potato casserole with aluminum foil then bake for 45 minutes.

7. When the liquid mixture is set, remove the sweet potato casserole from the oven.

8. Serve and enjoy warm.

Each serving contains 219 Calories, 5.5 g Sugar, 15.9 g Net Carbs, 12.4 g Fats, 12.8 g Protein.

Recipe 20: Simple Baked Beans

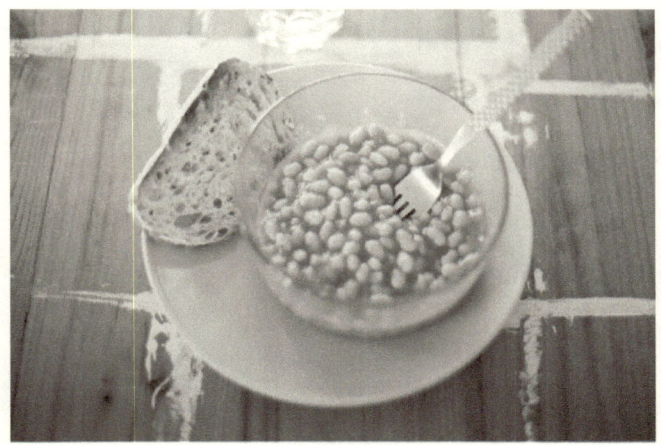

Baked bean is one of the beneficial foods for a pregnant woman. Besides providing fiber and protein, beans are also high of key nutrients such as zinc, calcium, and iron. If you are not a beans lover before, you can start with this baked bean recipe. Enjoy the baked beans with toasted whole grain bread, baked potato, or low carbs waffle.

Yield: 2

Preparation Time: 30 minutes

Ingredient List:

- ¾ cup cooked beans
- ½ tbsp. olive oil
- ¼ cup chopped onion
- 2 tsp. minced garlic
- ¾ tbsp. low sodium soy sauce
- ¾ tsp. mustard

HHHHHHHHHHHHHHHHHHHHHHHHHHHHHHHHHHH

Procedure:

1. Preheat an oven to 350°F then coat a baking dish with cooking spray.

2. Preheat a skillet over medium heat then pour olive oil into it.

3. Once it is hot, stir in chopped onion and minced garlic then sauté until translucent and aromatic.

4. Add beans to the skillet then season with low sodium soy sauce and mustard.

5. Transfer the beans to the prepared baking dish then spread evenly.

6. Bake for 20 minutes then once it is done, remove from the oven and transfer to a serving dish.

7. Serve and enjoy.

Each serving contains 124 Calories, 2.8 g Sugar, 12.4 g Net Carbs, 7.9 g Fats, 3.5 g Protein

Chapter III – Lunch Ideas

HHHHHHHHHHHHHHHHHHHHHHHHHHHHHHHHHHH

Recipe 21: Pulled Pork

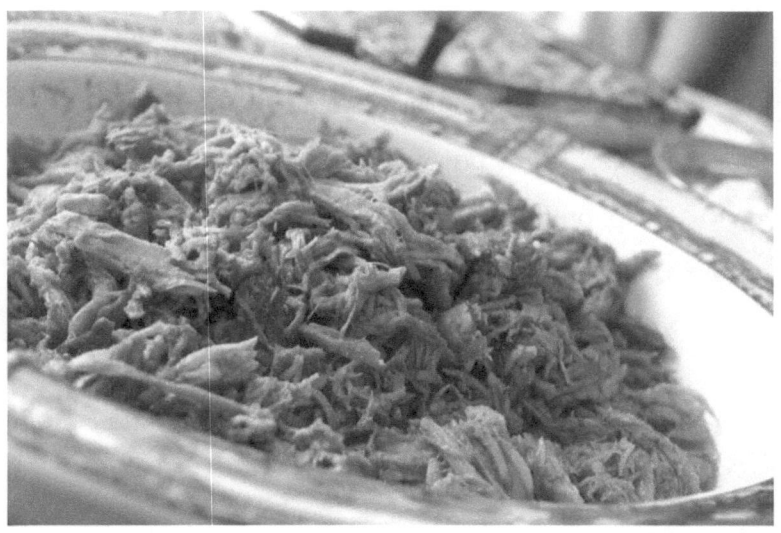

Pulled pork is a great choice. Not only the pregnant woman, but also the whole family can enjoy this delicious food. You can cook this pulled pork the night before and reheat it for a few minutes. It can be served with a slice of whole grain bread, whole grain tacos, a half-cup of cooked brown rice, or just eat it just the way it is. Having vegetable salads as a side dish is also a good alternative.

Yield: 2

Preparation Time: 3 hours 30 minutes

Ingredient List:

- 1 lb. pork roast
- ½ tsp. black pepper
- ¾ tsp. red chili flakes
- 1-¼ tsp. garlic powder
- ¾ tsp. onion powder
- ¾ tsp. mustard
- ¾ cup low sodium chicken broth

HHHHHHHHHHHHHHHHHHHHHHHHHHHHHHHHHHH

Procedure:

1. Preheat an oven to 450°F then coat a baking dish with cooking spray.

2. Combine black pepper with red chili flakes, garlic powder, onion powder, and mustard.

3. Rub the pork roast with the spice mixture then place the pork in the prepared baking dish.

4. Bake the pork for an hour.

5. After an hour, reduce the heat to 350°F then pour low sodium chicken broth over the pork.

6. Return to the oven then cover with aluminum foil.

7. Bake the pork again for about 2 hours or until the pork is tender.

8. Once it is done, take the pork out from the oven then let it cool for a few minutes.

9. Wait until the pork is cool or warm then using a fork shred the pork.

10. Transfer to a serving dish then enjoy.

Each serving contains 373 Calories, 0.9 g Sugar, 3.1 g Net Carbs, 16.5 g Fats, 49.9 g Protein

Recipe 22: Chicken Cucumber Salads

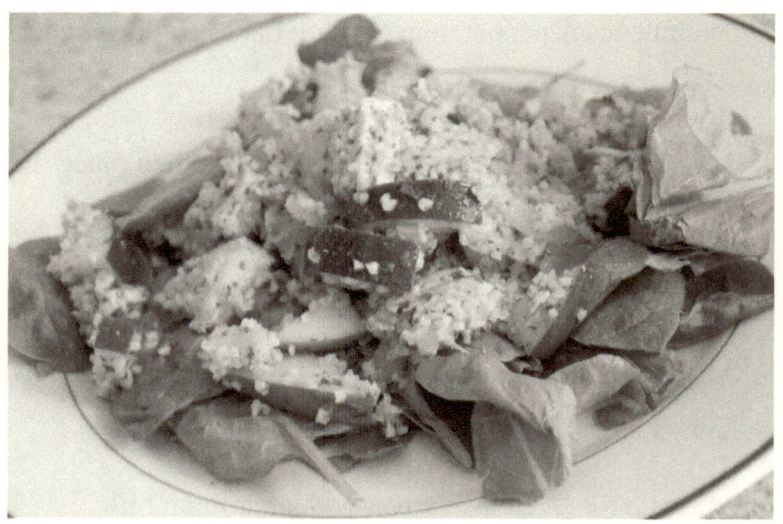

This dish is a great choice for a pregnant woman. Chicken, that is high in protein and fats can be a great source of energy without increasing the sugar level in the blood. Cucumber, as the partner for chicken in this dish, is absolutely healthy. The high fiber content in cucumber will ensure the digestive system runs well while the high water content will avoid the pregnant woman from dehydration. Enjoy this dish with a half bowl of cooked brown rice.

Yield: 1

Preparation Time: 5 Minutes

Ingredient List:

- 1 cup chopped cooked chicken
- 1 medium cucumber
- ½ tbsp. peanut butter
- ¾ tsp. low sodium soy sauce
- ½ tsp. sesame oil
- ¼ tsp. ginger
- ¼ tsp. minced garlic

HHHHHHHHHHHHHHHHHHHHHHHHHHHHHHHHHH

Procedure:

1. First, prepare the dressing,

2. Place a tbsp. of peanut butter in a bowl then add soy sauce, sesame oil, ginger, and minced garlic. Mix well then set aside.

3. Cut the cucumber into cubes then place in a salad bowl—discard the seeds.

4. Add chopped chicken to the bowl the mix with the cucumber cubes.

5. Drizzle the dressing on top then serve immediately.

6. If you want to consume it later, cover the chicken and cucumber with plastic wrap then refrigerate.

7. Once you want to consume, take it out from the refrigerator then unwrap.

8. Drizzle the dressing on top then enjoy immediately.

Each serving contains 328 Calories, 5.9 g Sugar, 13.4 g Net Carbs, 10.9 g Fats, 44.8 g Protein

Recipe 23: Roasted Mixed Vegetables

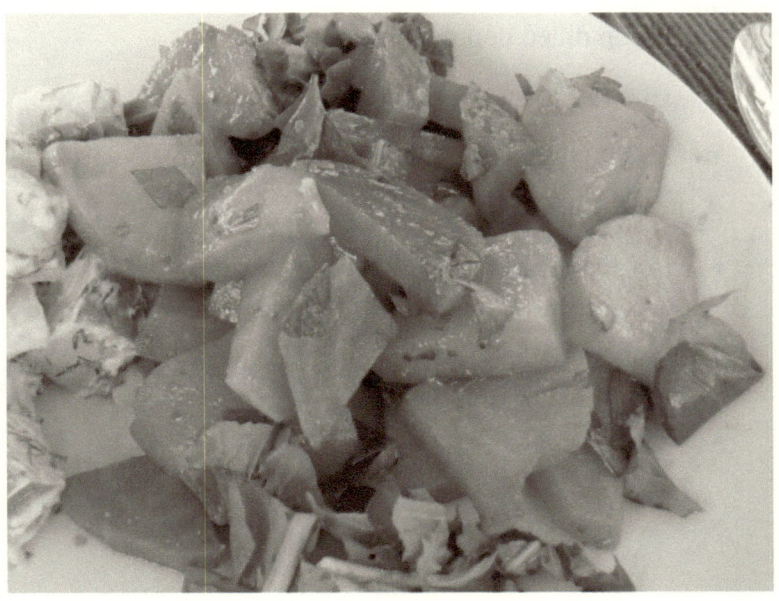

Roasted vegetables are not only healthy but also tasty. Beta-carotene, vitamin C, Potassium, and folic acid are good nutrients that can be found in vegetables. Choose the freshest vegetables you can find for this recipe, they are good for a pregnant woman. Not only it is healthier, but fresh vegetables also offer a tastier taste. Eat roasted vegetables with grilled or sautéed meat for a complete nutrient consumption.

Yield: 4

Preparation Time: 50 minutes

Ingredient List:

- 1-cup butternut squash cubes
- ½ cup diced bell peppers
- 1-cup sweet potato cubes
- ½ cup chopped onion
- ¾ tbsp. thyme
- 1-½ tbsp. rosemary
- 3 tbsp. olive oil
- 1-½ tbsp. balsamic vinegar
- ½ tsp. pepper

HHHHHHHHHHHHHHHHHHHHHHHHHHHHHHHHHHHHHH

Procedure:

1. Preheat an oven to 475°F then coat a baking dish with cooking spray.

2. Place butternut squash, bell pepper, potato cubes, and chopped onion in the prepared baking dish.

3. Sprinkle thyme, rosemary, and pepper then drizzle olive oil and balsamic vinegar over the vegetables. Toss to combine.

4. Roast the vegetables for about 45 minutes or until the vegetables are tender enough.

5. Once it is done, transfer to a serving dish then serve.

6. Enjoy.

Each serving contains 127 Calories, 2.8 g Sugar, 8.4 g Net Carbs, 10.7 g Fats, 0.9 g Protein

Recipe 24: Chicken Tomato Taco

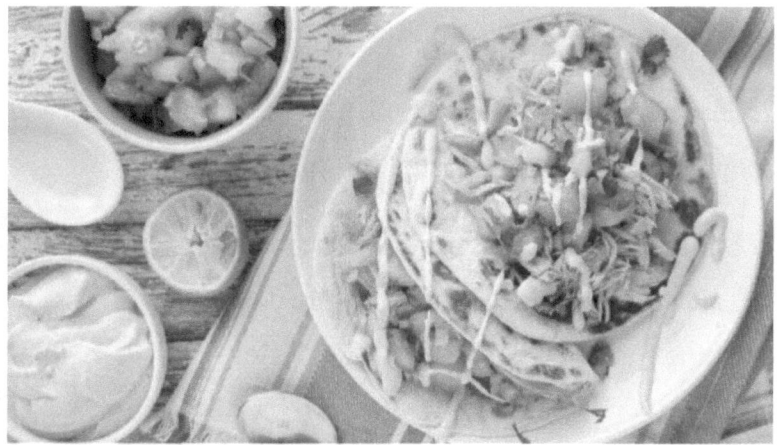

Taco is a practical lunch. The filling can be prepared ahead of time and stored in the refrigerator. Once you want to consume it, you just have to microwave it for a few seconds then the filling will taste a great as before. You can also make lots of variation for the filling. Not only chicken, but beef, pork, tuna, or mushroom can also be a good option for a taco filling. Don't forget to choose whole grain taco for a lower carbs choice.

Yield: 1

Preparation Time: 20 Minutes

Ingredient List:

- ½ cup chopped cooked chicken
- ½ tsp. olive oil
- 1 tsp. minced garlic
- ¼ tsp. pepper
- 2 tbsp. diced tomato
- 1 whole grains tortilla
- Fresh celery, for garnish

HHHHHHHHHHHHHHHHHHHHHHHHHHHHHHHHHHH

Procedure:

1. Preheat a skillet over medium heat then pour olive oil into it.

2. Once it is hot, stir in minced garlic then sauté until aromatic.

3. Add chopped chicken to the skillet then season with pepper. Stir well then remove from heat.

4. Place a tortilla on a flat surface then drop the chicken in the center of the tortilla.

5. Add diced tomatoes on the chicken then fold the tortilla.

6. Bake the tortilla if you want or just enjoy it right away.

7. Garnish with fresh celery if you like.

8. Enjoy!

Each serving contains 276 Calories, 5.1 g Sugar, 21 g Net Carbs, 11.5 g Fats, 22.8 g Protein

Recipe 25: Mushroom Beef Stew

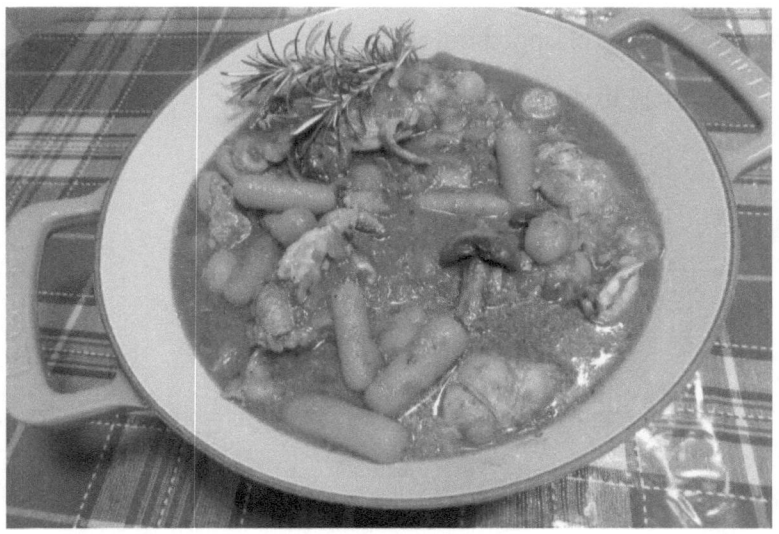

Mushroom has been known as a great antioxidant. Besides that, a mushroom is also a great option for a pregnant woman for it contains fiber, iron, and lots of vitamins. A combination of mushroom and beef does not only serve beneficial nutrients but also has a scrumptious taste. Moreover, additional vegetables in this dish will make this dish even more irresistible.

Yield: 4

Preparation Time: 4 hours

Ingredient List:

- 1 medium carrot
- ½ cup chopped onion
- 1 ½ lb. beef
- 1 cup chopped mushroom
- 1-½ cups beef broth
- ¾ tsp. thyme
- ½ cup green peas

HHHHHHHHHHHHHHHHHHHHHHHHHHHHHHHHHHH

Procedure:

1. Cut the beef into slices then place in a slow cooker.

2. Peel the carrots then cut into thick slices. Stir in the sliced carrot into the slow cooker pot.

3. Next, add green peas, onion, and mushroom then pour beef broth over the beef.

4. Add thyme then cover the slow cooker with its lid properly.

5. Select the low heat menu then set the cooking time to 8 hours or 4 hours on high heat.

6. Once it is done, open the slow cooker then add peas to the stew. Quickly stir the stew until then peas are well combined.

7. Transfer to a serving dish then enjoy.

Each serving contains 369 Calories, 4.4 g Sugar, 9.4 g Net Carbs, 11.1 g Fats, 54.9 g Protein

Recipe 26: Delicious Pork Loaf

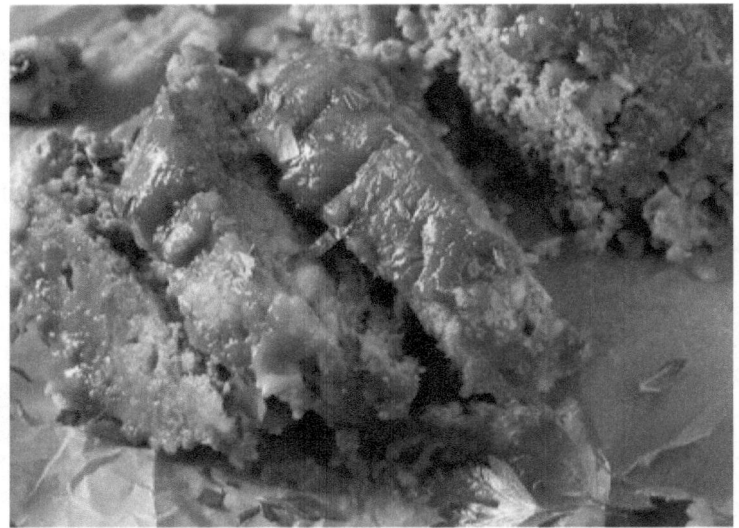

The great things about this menu are it is practical to cook and carry, can make you full easily, is nutritious, and can be stored for later. If you don't like pork, you can change it into meat, lamb, chicken, or even tuna.

Yield: 4

Preparation Time: 1 hour 10 Minutes

Ingredient List:

- 1 lb. ground beef
- 2 tsp. minced garlic
- ½ tsp. pepper
- ¾ cup chopped onion
- 1 organic egg
- ½ cup rolled oats

HHHHHHHHHHHHHHHHHHHHHHHHHHHHHHHHHHH

Procedure:

1. Preheat an oven to 375°F then prepare a baking sheet. Set aside.

2. Place ground beef and oats in a food processor.

3. Add minced garlic, pepper, onion, and egg then process until smooth.

4. Prepare a sheet of aluminum foil then place the beef mixture on it.

5. Shape the mixture into a log then tightly wrap with the aluminum foil.

6. Place the log on the prepared baking sheet then bake for about an hour.

7. Once it is done, remove from the oven and let it sit for a few minutes until warm.

8. Unwrap the log then cut into thick slices.

9. Serve and enjoy.

Each serving contains 274 Calories, 1.1 g Sugar, 9.2 g Net Carbs, 8.9 g Fats, 37.4 g Protein

Recipe 27: Spicy Beef Lettuce Wraps

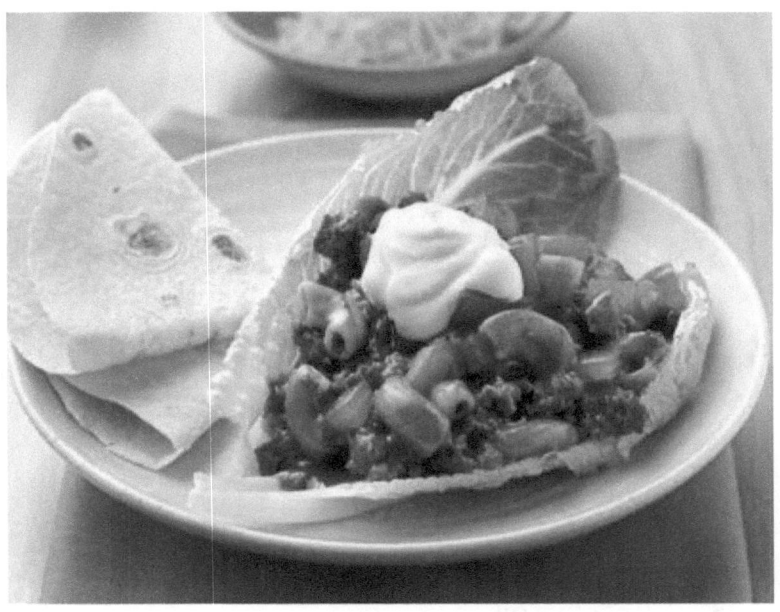

There is no reason for a pregnant woman to skip their lunch. A pregnant woman doesn't only eat for herself but also for the baby. This dish offers a practicability and delicacy at the same time. The filling can be made in advance and stored in the refrigerator. Once you want to consume it, just microwave for a few seconds then wrap with fresh lettuce. Enjoy this on the go lunch and get the essential benefits.

Yield: 1

Preparation Time: 10 Minutes

Ingredient List:

- ¼ cup boneless beef
- ¼ cup chopped green beans
- 2 tbsp. chopped onion
- 1 tsp. minced garlic
- ½ tsp. red chili flakes
- 1-tbsp. paprika
- ¼ tsp. ginger
- ½ cup low sodium beef broth
- ¾ tsp. soy sauce
- 1-tbsp. oyster sauce
- ¼ tsp. pepper
- 1-tsp. olive oil
- ½ handful fresh lettuce

HHHHHHHHHHHHHHHHHHHHHHHHHHHHHHHHHHHH

Procedure:

1. Preheat a skillet over medium heat then pour olive oil into it.

2. Once it is hot, stir in minced garlic and chopped onion then sauté until wilted and aromatic.

3. Cut the beef into slices then add to the skillet. Sauté until wilted.

4. Pour low sodium beef broth over the beef then add green beans, chili flakes, and paprika.

5. Season with ginger, soy sauce, oyster sauce, and pepper then cook until the beef broth has reduced to half.

6. Once it is done and the beef is tender, remove from heat.

7. Place fresh lettuce on a plate then drop the cooked beef and vegetables on top.

8. Serve and enjoy.

Each serving contains 331 Calories, 2.7 g Sugar, 11.4 g Net Carbs, 26.9 g Fats, 12.9 g Protein

Recipe 28: Savory Shrimps Soup

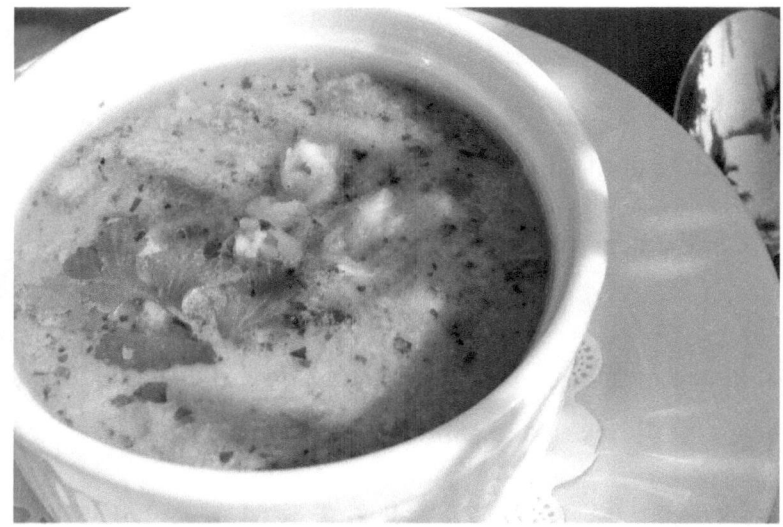

Shrimps soup is everyone's favorite. It is not only easy to make but also delicious. Other than that, shrimp is a great source of protein. For sure, it is very good for a pregnant woman. Shrimps only need a short period of time to be cooked. So, if you want to keep the original savory taste of the shrimps, make sure that you stir in them at the last minute.

Yield: 1

Preparation Time: 20 Minutes

Ingredient List:

- ¼ lb. fresh shrimps
- 1 medium carrot
- 1 tsp. sliced garlic
- 1 tsp. sliced shallot
- ¼ tsp. pepper
- ¼ tsp. ginger
- ½ tsp. red chili flakes
- 1 tbsp. lemon juice
- 2 tbsp. coconut milk
- ¼ cup water

HHHHHHHHHHHHHHHHHHHHHHHHHHHHHHHHHHHH

Procedure:

1. Peel carrot then cut into slices.

2. Place the carrot in a pot then pour water into the pot. Bring to boil.

3. Once it is boiled, stir in sliced garlic, sliced shallots, pepper, ginger, red chili flakes, and lemon juice into the pot. Stir well.

4. Add shrimps and coconut milk into the pot then bring to a simmer.

5. Once the shrimps are pink, quickly remove from heat then transfer to a serving dish.

6. Serve and enjoy warm.

Each serving contains 243 Calories, 4.5 g Sugar, 12 g Net Carbs, 9.3 g Fats, 27.5 g Protein

Recipe 29: Healthy Chicken Broccoli

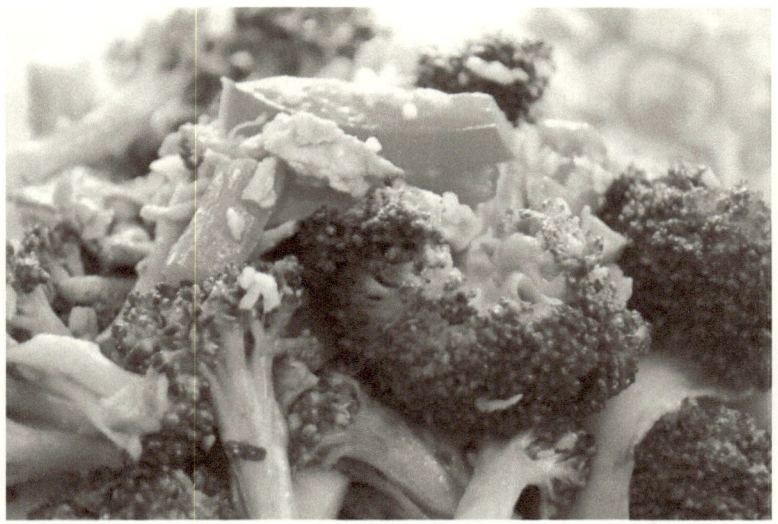

As the source of antioxidant, broccoli is a kind of vegetable that must be consumed by a pregnant woman. Besides that, it also offers lots of benefits for both the expectant woman and the baby such as healthier pregnancy, smoother skin, and stronger immunity. Don't overcook the broccoli to keep the crispy texture. Also, don't reheat it. Broccoli is best to be consumed fresh.

Yield: 1

Preparation Time: 10 Minutes

Ingredient List:

- ¼ lb. boneless chicken
- ½ cup broccoli florets
- ¼ cup chopped leek
- 1-tsp. olive oil
- 2 tsp. minced garlic
- ½ tsp. pepper
- 1-tsp. low sodium soy sauce
- ½ cup water

HHHHHHHHHHHHHHHHHHHHHHHHHHHHHHHHHHHH

Procedure:

1. Preheat a skillet over medium heat then pour olive oil into it.

2. Once the oil is hot, stir in minced garlic then sauté until lightly brown and aromatic.

3. Pour water over the chicken then cook until the water is absorbed into the chicken.

4. Add broccoli florets and leek into the skillet then drizzle soy sauce on top.

5. Season with pepper then stir well.

6. Cook until the vegetables are just wilted then transfer to a serving dish.

7. Serve and enjoy.

Each serving contains 298 Calories, 1.8 g Sugar, 9.2 g Net Carbs, 13.4 g Fats, 35.2 g Protein

Recipe 30: Baked Pork Fritter

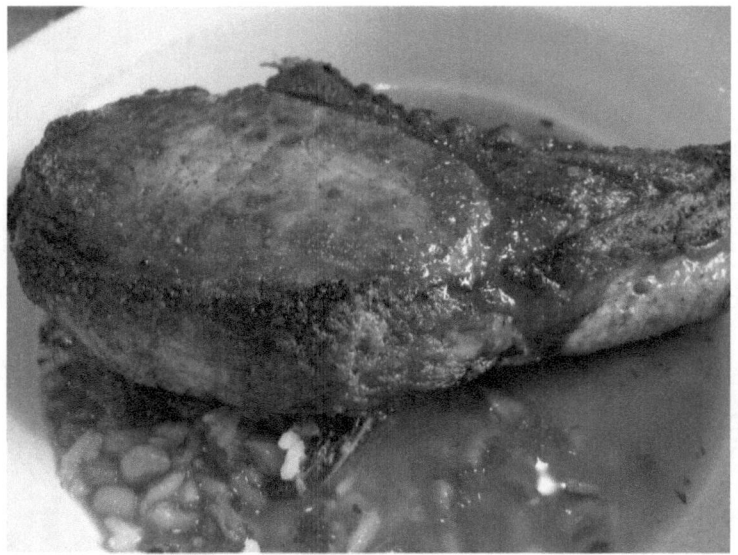

It is important to put in mind that busy days should not make you skip your meal. For a pregnant woman, the nutrient is the most important thing. This dish is an on the go lunch that you can be eaten during your busy days. Keep it in your lunch box and have your lunch even you are on a busy work or trip. If you don't like pork, you can substitute it with chicken, beef, or fish. Besides that, you can also add mushroom, sausage, or bacon, to enhance the taste.

Yield: 2

Preparation Time: 25 Minutes

Ingredient List:

- ½ lb. ground pork
- ¼ tsp. pepper
- ¼ cup chopped onion
- 2 tsp. minced garlic
- ½ tsp. thyme
- ½ tsp. coriander
- ½ tsp. cumin

HHHHHHHHHHHHHHHHHHHHHHHHHHHHHHHHHHH

Procedure:

1. Preheat an oven to 400°F then line a baking sheet with aluminum foil.

2. Place all ingredients in a food processor then process to combine.

3. Shape the mixture into medium fritter then arrange on the prepared baking sheet.

4. Bake the pork fritters for about 15 minutes until the fritters are lightly brown.

5. Once the fritters are done, remove from the oven then transfer to a serving dish.

6. Enjoy!

Each serving contains 175 Calories, 0.7 g Sugar, 2.8 g Net Carbs, 4.2 g Fats, 30.2 g Protein

Chapter IV – Dinner Ideas

HHHHHHHHHHHHHHHHHHHHHHHHHHHHHHHHHHHHH

Recipe 31: Steamed Fish with Green Chili

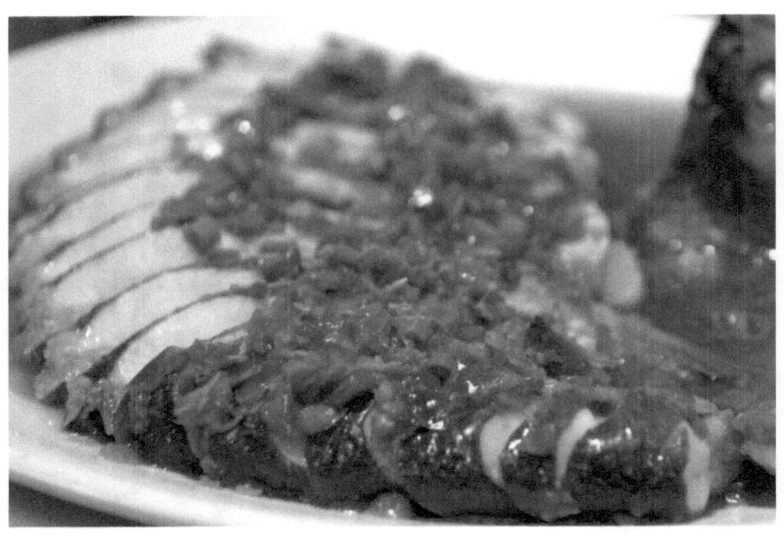

Steamed fish is considered as healthy food as it is completely oil-free. You can use any kinds of fish for the recipe. However, you have to ensure that the fish you use is fresh. This dish is designed especially for the spicy lovers. However, if you don't like a spicy taste, you can just simply skip the green chili. Or, if you like not too spicy taste, you can reduce the amount of green chili in this recipe.

Yield: 2

Preparation Time: 30 minutes

Ingredient List:

- 2 medium fresh fish
- 3 cloves garlic
- 4 shallots
- ½ tsp. ginger
- 1 bay leaf
- 1-inch galangal
- ¼ cup green chili

HHHHHHHHHHHHHHHHHHHHHHHHHHHHHHHHHHHHH

Procedure:

1. Preheat a steamer then prepare a heatproof dish.

2. Place garlic, shallot, and green chili in a food processor then pulse to combine.

3. Rub the fish with the spice mixture then place in the prepared dish.

4. Add galangal and bay leaf to the dish then steam for about 30 minutes.

5. Once it is done, remove the fish from steamer then serve.

6. Enjoy warm.

Each serving contains 166 Calories, 2.3 g Sugar, 16.1 g Net Carbs, 1.3 g Fats, 21.8 g Protein

Recipe 32: Buttery Beef Steak

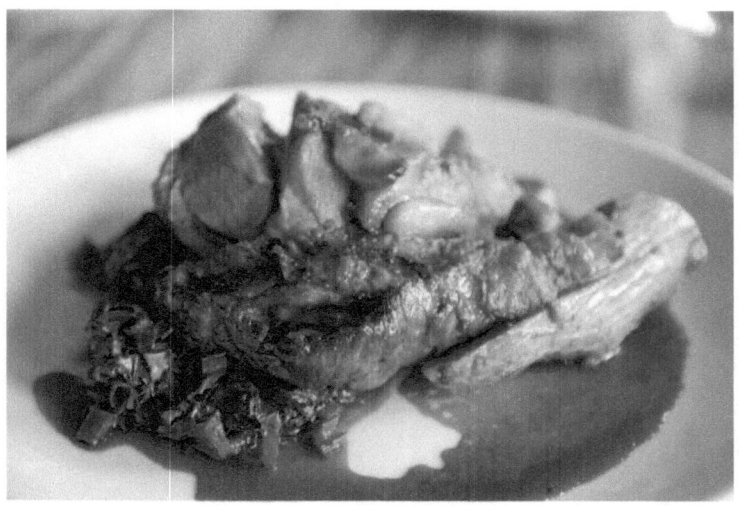

Beefsteak, no one can deny the delicacy of a beefsteak. Unlike other steaks that may need a longer period of time to be prepared, this beefsteak is ready in a few minutes. This is absolutely a plus. The best thing about this dish is that the doneness of the steak that you like. Grill the steak over medium heat then determine your desired doneness and enjoy warm. For a perfect result, have this beefsteak with roasted vegetables as the source of vitamins and potatoes as the source of carbohydrates. Pay attention that it is not recommended for a pregnant woman to eat rare meat with the fear that there must be some bacteria or viruses that may attack the baby.

Yield: 2

Preparation Time: 15 minutes

Ingredient List:

- 1 lb. sirloin
- 3 tbsp. almond butter
- 1 tsp. minced garlic
- ½ tsp. black pepper

HHHHHHHHHHHHHHHHHHHHHHHHHHHHHHHHHHH

Procedure:

1. Preheat a grill over medium heat.

2. Place the almond butter in a saucepan then preheat over medium heat.

3. Once the butter is melted, stir in minced garlic then sauté until wilted and aromatic. Set aside.

4. Sprinkle black pepper over the sirloin, and then grill until it reaches your desired doneness. Around 5 minutes to reach medium-rare doneness and around 9 minutes for medium one.

5. Once it is done, transfer to a serving dish then quickly drizzle the melted butter over the steak.

6. Serve and enjoy warm.

Each serving contains 388 Calories, 1.1 g Sugar, 5.3 g Net Carbs, 21.5 g Fats, 44 g Protein

Recipe 33: Pork Satay in Tomato Sauce

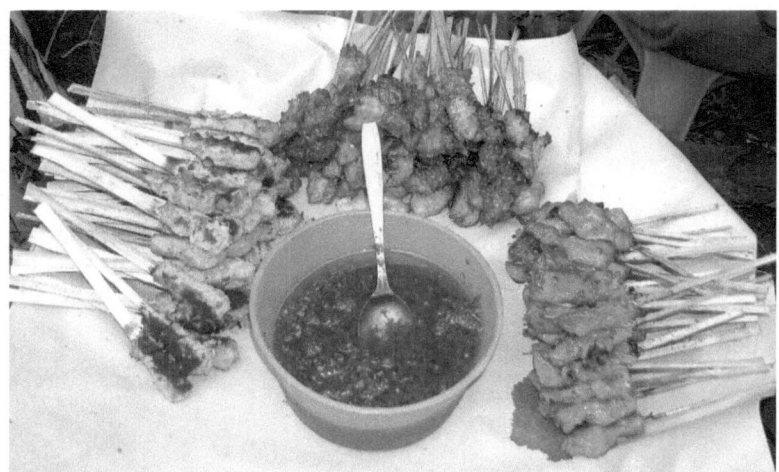

Satay is sometimes unsafe for a pregnant woman. However, it can be ensured that this pork satay is completely safe. This satay is seasoned with traditional herbs to give special touch for this dish. It is also cooked over medium heat until tender and well done. The grilling process in this pork satay is just to give the smell of smoke to this dish.

Yield: 2

Preparation Time: 1 hour 30 minutes

Ingredient List:

- ½ lb. pork lean
- 1 tsp. minced garlic
- 1-tsp. coriander
- 1 bay leaf
- 2 kefir lime leaves
- 2 cups water
- ½ tsp. olive oil
- 1cup tomato puree
- 2 tbsp. chopped onion
- ½ tsp. nutmeg
- ½ tsp. pepper
- ½ cup low sodium beef broth

HHHHHHHHHHHHHHHHHHHHHHHHHHHHHHHHHH

Procedure:

1. Cut the pork lean into cubes then place in a pot

2. Season with minced garlic, coriander, bay leaves, and kefir lime leaves then pour water into the pot. Bring to boil.

3. Once it is boiled, reduce the heat then cook until the pork is tender. Remove from heat.

4. Let the cooked pork cool then prick with wooden skewers.

5. Preheat a grill to medium heat.

6. Meanwhile, preheat a skillet then pour olive oil into it.

7. Once it is hot, stir in chopped onion into the skillet then sauté until translucent and aromatic.

8. Pour tomato puree into the skillet then season with pepper and nutmeg.

9. Add low sodium beef broth then bring to boil.

10. Once it is boiled, remove from heat then set aside.

11. When the grill is hot, place the pork satay on the grill then grill until a bit brown.

12. Once it is done, place the pork satay on a serving platter then drizzle tomato sauce over the pork.

13. Serve and enjoy.

Each serving contains 299 Calories, 7.9 g Sugar, 20.9 g Net Carbs, 13.3 g Fats, 29.2 g Protein

Recipe 34: Mixed Cauliflower Curry

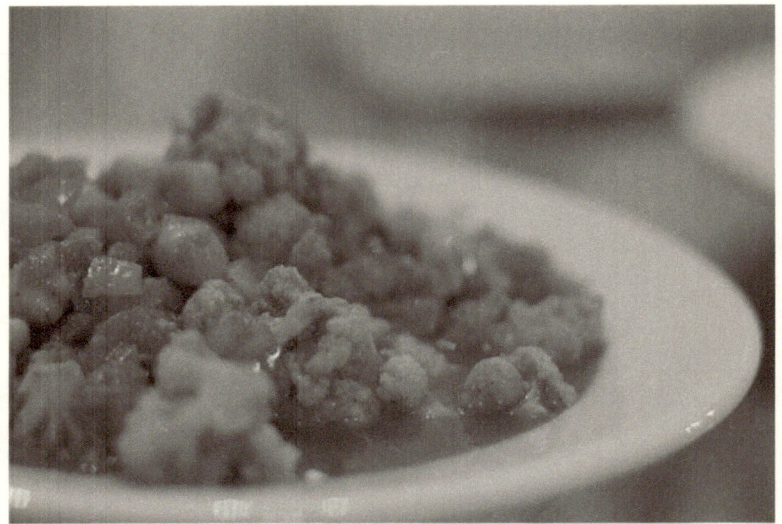

Cauliflower is one of the vegetables that are good to be consumed during pregnancy. Besides antioxidant, cauliflower also serves many minerals that are good for the pregnant women, such as selenium, zinc, phosphorus, and sodium. For it is also high fiber and low in cholesterol, cauliflower is good to be consumed every day. To enhance the taste, add other vegetables to this recipe.

Yield: 1

Preparation Time: 20 minutes

Ingredient List:

- ½ cup cauliflower florets
- ¼ cup green peas
- ¼ cup sliced carrots
- ¼ cup chopped onion
- 1 tsp. minced garlic
- ¼ tsp. ginger
- ¼ tsp. olive oil
- ¾ tsp. cumin
- ½ tsp. coriander
- ¼ tsp. cumin
- ½ tsp. turmeric
- ¾ tsp. cayenne pepper
- 1 tsp. chopped green chili
- 2 tbsp. chopped tomato
- 2 cups water

HHHHHHHHHHHHHHHHHHHHHHHHHHHHHHHHHHH

Procedure:

1. Preheat a skillet over medium heat then pour olive oil into it.

2. Once it is hot, stir in minced garlic and onion then sauté until wilted and aromatic.

3. Add ginger, cumin, turmeric, cayenne pepper, and green chili to the skillet then stir in sliced carrot, green peas, and cauliflower florets. Sauté until wilted and seasoned.

4. Pour water over the vegetables then bring to boil.

5. Once it is boiled, reduce the heat and cook until the vegetables are tender.

6. Transfer to a serving bowl then serve warm.

Each serving contains 126 Calories, 4.7 g Sugar, 18.6 g Net Carbs, 4.7 g Fats, 4.7 g Protein

Recipe 35: Simple Kale Garlic

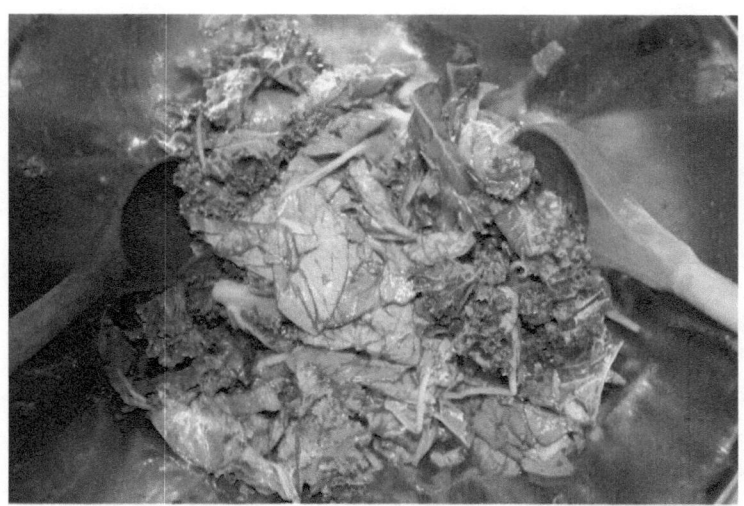

Kale is a super food that is good to be included in an expectant mother's diet. This green vegetable is loaded with fiber, calcium, vitamin C, and vitamin A. For sure, an expectant mother needs those nutrients. Some people say that kale sometimes smells like sulfur. However, with the help of garlic, it can be reduced. If you like a spicy taste, you can add a tsp. of red chili flakes to this dish.

Yield: 1

Preparation Time: 15 minutes

Ingredient List:

- 2 cups chopped kale
- 1-tbsp. olive oil
- 2 tsp. minced garlic
- ¾ cup water

HHHHHHHHHHHHHHHHHHHHHHHHHHHHHHHHHHH

Procedure:

1. Preheat a skillet over medium heat then sauté kale in oil together with the minced garlic.

2. Once the kale is wilted, pour water into the skillet then bring to boil.

3. Once it is boiled, reduce the heat then cook until the kale is tender.

4. Transfer to a serving dish then serve.

5. Enjoy right away.

Each serving contains 194 Calories, 0.1 g Sugar, 15.9 g Net Carbs, 14 g Fats, 4.4 g Protein

Recipe 36: Roasted Chicken with Potato and Tomato

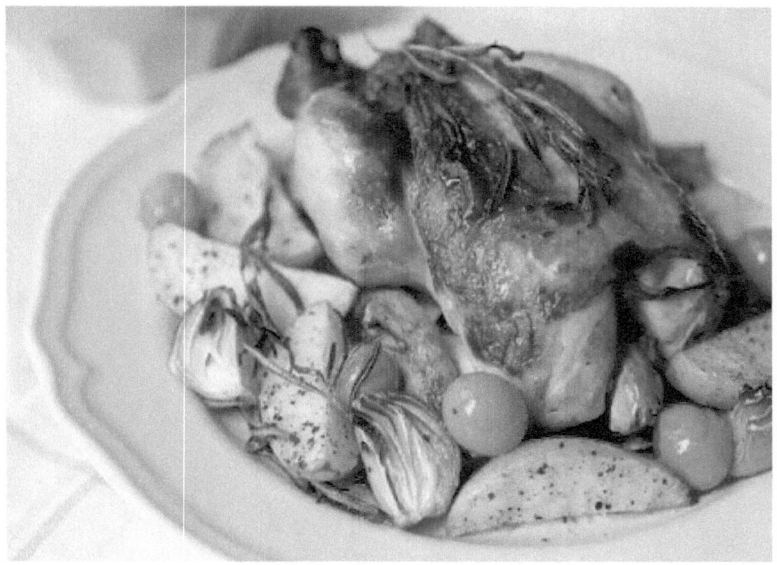

The reasons why this dish becomes a great choice for dinner that it is simple to prepare and delicious. Chicken is also healthier because it contains minerals, vitamins, and proteins that will help the baby to grow better. Things that should be concerned relating to this dish is the doneness of the chicken. Make sure that you have completely cooked the chicken before consuming it. Also, choose organic chicken whenever possible because, surely, organic chicken is healthier than the non-organic one.

Yield: 4

Preparation Time: 55 Minutes

Ingredient List:

- 1 medium whole chicken
- 2-½ tbsp. olive oil
- 2 tbsp. thyme
- 1 ¼ tsp. black pepper
- 1 lb. small potatoes
- ½ lb. tomatoes

HHHHHHHHHHHHHHHHHHHHHHHHHHHHHHHHHHHH

Procedure:

1. Preheat an oven to 425°F then lines a baking dish with aluminum foil.

2. Combine olive oil with thyme and black pepper then mix well.

3. Cut the small potatoes and tomatoes into halves then sprinkle on the bottom of the prepared baking dish.

4. Place the chicken on the potatoes with the meaty side down.

5. Brush the chicken with the olive oil mixture then drizzle the remaining oil mixture over the potatoes and tomatoes.

6. Roast the chicken for 45 minutes or until the chicken is done.

7. Remove the chicken from the oven then transfer to a serving dish together with the potatoes and tomatoes.

8. Enjoy warm.

Each serving contains 219 Calories, 2.8 g Sugar, 21.3 g Net Carbs, 11.6 g Fats, 7.9 g Protein

Recipe 37: Boiled Eggs in Red Thick Gravy

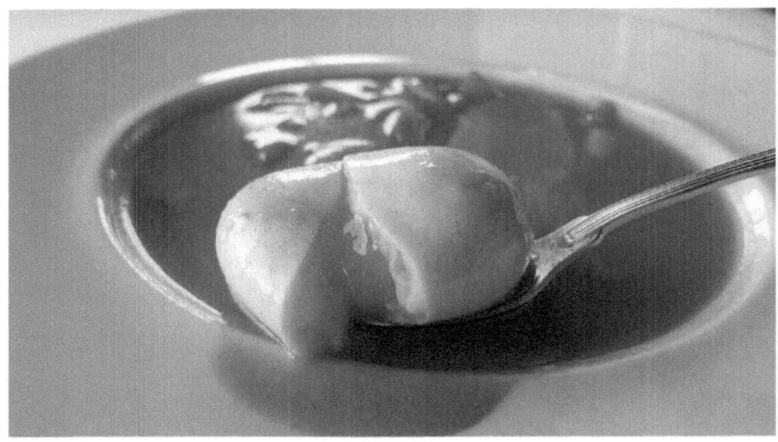

The egg is packaged with nutrients that make it count as a healthy food. Protein, mineral, and fats are the beneficial nutrients that are needed by a pregnant woman. Since egg contains those nutrients, it is good to include egg in your pregnancy. Seasoned with complete herbs, this dish serves a scrumptious taste that you cannot imagine. If you like crunchy sensation, you can fry the boiled eggs before adding them to the gravy. You can also substitute the chicken eggs with other eggs if you like.

Yield: 4

Preparation Time: 30 minutes

Ingredient List:

- 8 boiled eggs
- 1-tsp. canola oil
- 2 tsp. minced garlic
- 2 tsp. sliced shallot
- 2 tbsp. chopped red chili
- 1 bay leaf
- 1-inch galangal
- 1-½ cups water
- ½ cup coconut milk
- ¼ cup tomato puree

HHHHHHHHHHHHHHHHHHHHHHHHHHHHHHHHHH

Procedure:

1. Preheat a skillet over medium heat then pour canola oil into it.

2. Once it is hot, stir in minced garlic and shallot then sauté until wilted and aromatic.

3. Add red chili, bay leaf, and galangal then pour water into the skillet.

4. Peel the eggs then place them in the skillet. Bring to boiled.

5. Once it is boiled, add the tomato puree then pour coconut milk. Bring to a simmer for approximately 5 minutes.

6. Transfer to a serving dish then enjoy.

Each serving contains 220 Calories, 3 g Sugar, 5.7 g Net Carbs, 17.2 g Fats, 12.3 g Protein

Recipe 38: Savory Shrimps Veggie

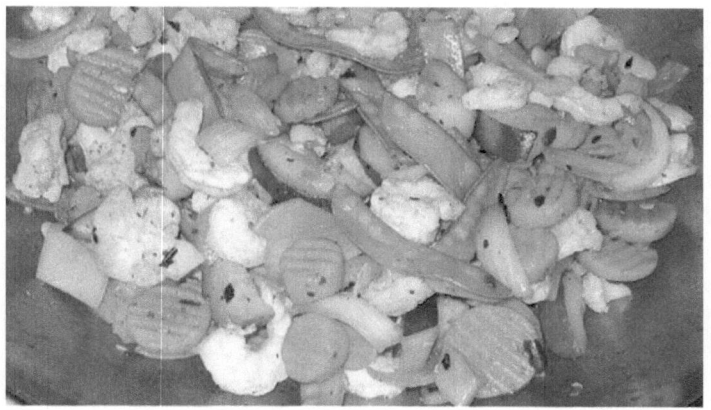

This food is loaded with vegetables, shrimps, and spices. It is a low carb but high in beneficial nutrients. You can mix the vegetables according to your preference. Also, you can add other kinds of seafood that you like. Whatever the ingredients are, as long as they are fresh and cooked well, this dish will taste delicious. Another good thing about this dish is that it doesn't need much time to cook. You only have to invest a few minutes of your time to serve this tempting dish on your dining table. Be cautious that all seafood that you eat should be cooked properly to avoid bacteria or virus contamination in your baby.

Yield: 1

Preparation Time: 15 Minutes

Ingredient List:

- ½ cup fresh shrimps
- ½ cup broccoli florets
- 1 medium carrot
- 1-tsp. olive oil
- 2 tbsp. chopped onion
- ¼ tsp. pepper
- ¼ tsp. nutmeg
- ½ tsp. oyster sauce
- 2 tbsp. tomato puree
- ¼ cup low sodium chicken broth

HHHHHHHHHHHHHHHHHHHHHHHHHHHHHHHHHH

Procedure:

1. Peel the shrimps then discard the head. Set aside.

2. Peel and cut the carrot into stick then also set aside.

3. Preheat a skillet over medium heat then sauté onion together with oil.

4. Add the peeled shrimps then sauté until the color changes into pink.

5. Stir in carrot and broccoli florets then season with pepper, nutmeg, and oyster sauce.

6. Pour water and tomato puree then bring to boil. Cook until the vegetables are tender but still crispy.

7. Once it is done, transfer to a serving dish then serve right away.

8. Enjoy.

Each serving contains 189 Calories, 6.3 g Sugar, 14.6 g Net Carbs, 6.1 g Fats, 21.1 g Protein

Recipe 39: Baked Salmon Black Pepper

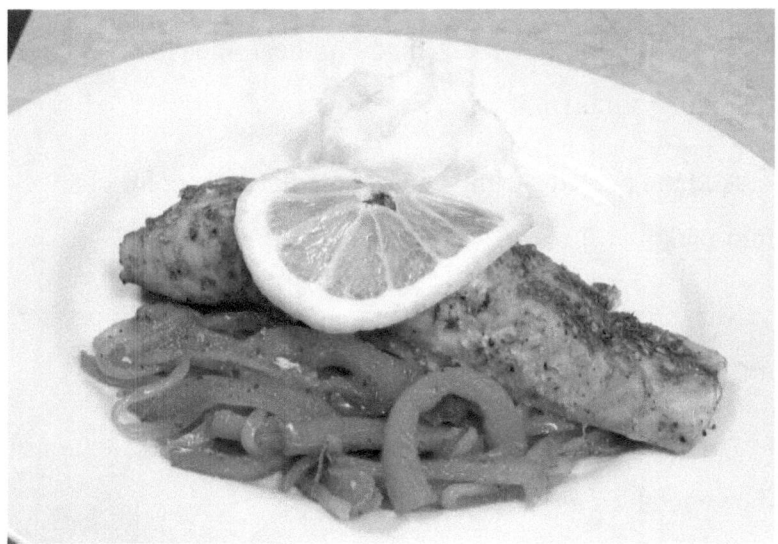

Salmon is high of omega-3 fatty acids that will lower the risk of preeclampsia and pre-term delivery. It is also a great source of vitamin B and protein. However, because raw fish sometimes contains bacteria, you have to ensure that you have cooked the salmon completely before eating them. Enjoy the baked salmon with vegetables or mix it with other fish. Some people prefer to consume baked salmon with sunny side up.

Yield: 2

Preparation Time: 20 minutes

Ingredient List:

- 1 lb. salmon steaks
- 2-½ tsp. olive oil
- 2 tsp. black pepper
- 1 tbsp. black sesame seeds

HHHHHHHHHHHHHHHHHHHHHHHHHHHHHHHHH

Procedure:

1. Preheat an oven to 350°F then lines a baking sheet with aluminum foil.

2. Brush the salmon with olive oil then sprinkle black pepper over the salmon.

3. Place the salmon on the prepared baking sheet then bake for approximately 15 minutes.

4. Take the salmon steaks out from the oven then flip them.

5. Brush the other sides with olive oil then sprinkle with black pepper and sesame seeds.

6. Return the salmon to the oven then bake again for another 15 minutes.

7. Once it is done, remove from the oven then transfer to a serving dish.

8. Serve and enjoy.

Each serving contains 371 Calories, 0 g Sugar, 2.4 g Net Carbs, 21 g Fats, 45 g Protein

Recipe 40: Pumpkin Soup

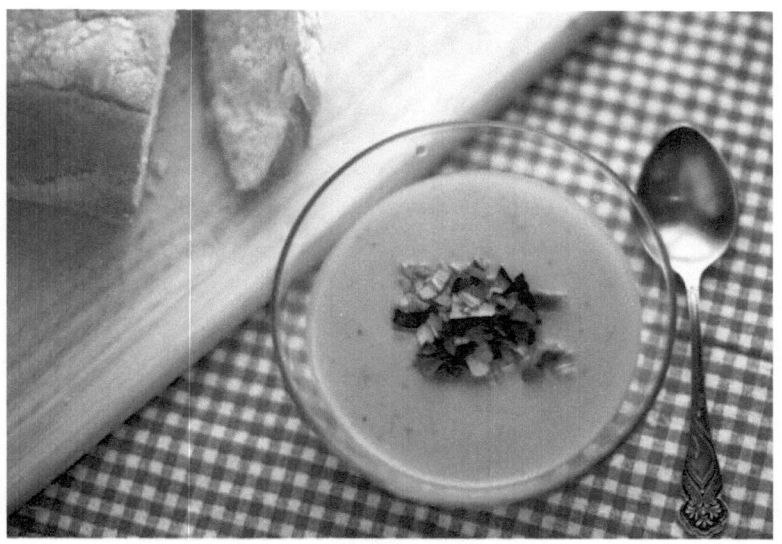

Known as a great source of vitamin A, pumpkin is one of the best ingredients that should be involved in a pregnant woman's meal. It reduces the blood sugar level in the body that automatically decreases the risk of having gestational diabetes. Besides that, pumpkin is also a high source of fiber that is much needed by an expectant mother to avoid constipation.

Yield: 2

Preparation Time: 20 minutes

Ingredient List:

- ¾ cup pumpkin puree
- ½ tsp. canola oil
- ¼ cup chopped onion
- ¼ cup chopped carrot
- 1-tbsp. celery stalk
- 2 cups low sodium chicken broth
- ¾ tsp. cinnamon
- ¼ tsp. pepper

HHHHHHHHHHHHHHHHHHHHHHHHHHHHHHHHHHHHH

Procedure:

1. Preheat a soup pot over medium heat then pour canola oil into the pot.

2. Once the oil is hot, stir in chopped onion and sauté until it is translucent and aromatic.

3. Add carrot and celery then stir until wilted.

4. Pour the chicken broth in the pot then season with cinnamon and pepper. Bring to a simmer.

5. Once it is done, remove from heat and let it sit for a few minutes until warm.

6. Using an immersion blender blend until smooth.

7. Transfer to a serving bowl then serve immediately.

Each serving contains 110 Calories, 5.7 g Sugar, 16.9 g Net Carbs, 2.4 g Fats, 5.5 g Protein.

About the Author

Angel Burns learned to cook when she worked in the local seafood restaurant near her home in Hyannis Port in Massachusetts as a teenager. The head chef took Angel under his wing and taught the young woman the tricks of the trade for cooking seafood. The skills she had learned at a young age helped her get accepted into Boston University's Culinary Program where she also minored in business administration.

Summers off from school meant working at the same restaurant but when Angel's mentor and friend retired as head chef, she took over after graduation and created classic and new dishes that delighted the diners. The restaurant flourished under Angel's culinary creativity and one customer developed more than an appreciation for Angel's food. Several months after taking over the position, the young woman met her future husband at work and they have been inseparable ever since. They still live in Hyannis Port with their two children and a cocker spaniel named Buddy.

Angel Burns turned her passion for cooking and her business acumen into a thriving e-book business. She has authored several successful books on cooking different types of dishes using simple ingredients for novices and experienced chefs alike. She is still head chef in Hyannis Port and says she will probably never leave!

Author's Afterthoughts

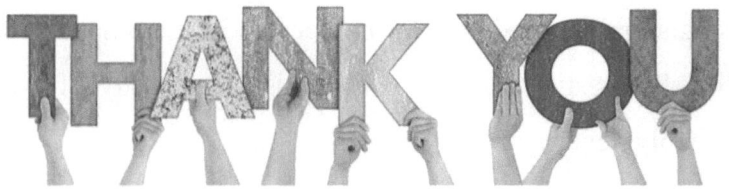

With so many books out there to choose from, I want to thank you for choosing this one and taking precious time out of your life to buy and read my work. Readers like you are the reason I take such passion in creating these books.

It is with gratitude and humility that I express how honored I am to become a part of your life and I hope that you take the same pleasure in reading this book as I did in writing it.

Can I ask one small favour? I ask that you write an honest and open review on Amazon of what you thought of the book. This will help other readers make an informed choice on whether to buy this book.

My sincerest thanks,

Angel Burns

If you want to be the first to know about news, new books, events and giveaways, subscribe to my newsletter by clicking the link below

https://angel-burns.gr8.com

or Scan QR-code

www.ingramcontent.com/pod-product-compliance
Lightning Source LLC
Chambersburg PA
CBHW020250290526
45784CB00003B/1185